Can You Walk Yet?

Book design by PenworthyLLC

ISBN: 978-09980616-0-3

Nothing is so healing as the human touch.

Bobby Fischer

Acknowledgments

I will be forever grateful and indebted to my husband, Glenn, who always supported me throughout my illness. To our son, Gary, and his wife, Janet, for giving up their jobs in New York and moving back to Blacksburg to help care for me; as well as to our daughter, Paula, and her late husband, Russell Lindsay, for their caring and loving support. To my late sister and brother-in-law, Madelyn and "Beanie" Oyer, and my late mother-in-law and father-in-law, Evelyn and Paul Buss. Without all of those family members, I would not have been able to overcome the terrible disease.

I cannot forget to mention my neighbors, church family and friends, who visited often to help me pass the time as I sat motionless in my chair.

Last, but certainly not least, I am indebted to Dean Kraft, who unfortunately passed away in October 2013. His special gift was phenomenal, and I was one of the fortunate who heard about him and had a family willing to take me to New York to see him every other week for more than a year.

Many thanks to Rachael Garrity for her expertise and help with editing and publishing this book.

Nelda Buss, August 2016

Foreword

This book was started 30 years ago. After contracting ALS, I quickly lost control of my arms and legs. I was fortunate that I could still control my head and neck muscles. I used a stick in my mouth, with a cup as a holder, to "type" on the keyboard of a computer at the kitchen table. I kept a diary of events. That is how this book evolved.

Chapter 1

My Early Life

Before January 1985, I lived a very normal life. I was the youngest in a family of three girls. My parents, Pearl and Paul Weidman, were very caring and hard-working individuals. We lived on a dairy farm just outside Bangor, a small town in eastern Pennsylvania. As my sisters and I grew up, we were expected to do our designated chores on our farm. As I became a teenager, I was feeding chickens and feeding and milking the cows, along with driving the tractor in the fields during the summer months. Driving the tractor was one job I didn't mind, since a good suntan was something that everyone liked at that age!

I must say, I think it would be good if everyone could grow up on the farm as I did. One learns to respect nature and the value of a dollar. I soon found out that if I ever wanted anything special, as I wanted a doll one time, I'd have to save my allowance and buy it myself. There just wasn't

1

enough income from the farm to buy unnecessary things. When my father needed equipment, he always bought used items, or he would fix up his old ones in order to survive.

Although I worked hard, I certainly can't say I didn't have any fun. I loved baby animals, whether it was a calf, a kitten, a pig or even mice. I surely could waste a lot of productive time fooling with them! I belonged to 4-H clubs for many years, and to the school band. I also attended Sunday School regularly.

I had many good times in 4-H. In fact, I met my husband, Glenn, at a 4-H meeting when I was very young. It always seemed that every boy I was interested in was never interested in me, and I never seemed to have any desire to go out on a date with the boys who were interested in me. Glenn was one of the latter.

My sister, Madelyn, had this long-time crush on Glenn's cousin, 'Skeeter.' Well, 'Skeeter' was a good-looking, smooth-talking young man. He called Madelyn one summer day to set up a date, saying he would be bringing Glenn Buss along for me and we would double date. Madelyn was overwhelmed with excitement. I was furious, but I agreed to go along with the scheme so Madelyn could go out on the date she had always dreamed about. Being the conniving Casanova that he was, 'Skeeter,' who never had any intention of going out with my sister, called her at the very last minute and canceled out on her, but assured her that Glenn would be at our doorstep shortly for me. I certainly was less than pleased with the situation, but there wasn't a whole heck of a lot I could do about it.

Our first date was in 1959, to a drive-in movie. (Glenn still kids me about that date. He says he was afraid I was going to fall out the door. I surely didn't want to get too close to him!) Then things changed. It seemed that after a year of dating, my desires changed, and I could never get enough of his dry wit and the wonderful feeling that everyone experiences when they are young and in love. On April 2, 1961, we eloped and were married in Bennettsville, SC.

I continued to live at home until Glenn finished his junior year at Penn State. We then purchased a one-bedroom 8` x 20` trailer. Since we were both from farms where we had been taught to save, we had put away money our whole lives and had enough to buy our first 'home.'

We lived in Schuylkill Haven that summer, while Glenn worked as a summer assistant county agent. That was not the most enjoyable summer I had ever experienced. I was pregnant, bored and homesick! Each weekday, I stayed home alone in the small, hot trailer and cleaned. We had no TV. I hated reading and knew no one. I insisted we travel two and a half hours to our childhood home every weekend. Glenn really wanted to stay 'home' after working all week, but he was good enough to understand my immature actions and helped wean me!

In September we moved our trailer to State College, Pennsylvania, where Glenn was to finish his under-graduate classes. We were then four hours from home, and by the end of October our first child was born. She was a healthy little girl, Paula, named after both of her grandfathers, who were named "Paul."

Glenn and I had a lot of adjustments to make that first year of marriage. We soon found out life wasn't always a bed of roses, like we had thought it would be before we were married. It seemed living with each other with full responsibility of a family was quite different. Once we weathered those stormy periods and gave birth to our second child, Gary, in 1964, we found ourselves adjusting to the typical American graduate student life.

Glenn was earning a whopping $2,400 a year as a graduate assistant in the Agronomy Department at Penn State. I earned $40 a month, our grocery money, baby-sitting at home. I must also mention that both his parents and mine did help us out with food from their farms. We also had space for a garden on our lot. By this time we had bought a larger trailer, 10` x 40`, and still were paying only $20 a month for lot rent. While we certainly had few luxuries, one of them was a poodle puppy, who was a gift from people whom we had helped seed their newly graded yard. Sheba, who lived to be 17 years old, turned out to be a very special dog to all of us.

Chapter 2

We Become Hokies

Finally, in August, 1967, Glenn graduated from Penn State with his doctorate degree in genetics. He landed his first job at the Virginia Polytechnic Institute (now known as Virginia Tech), Virginia's land grant university in Blacksburg. His starting salary was $11,000 a year. Well! We thought we were soon going to be rich! Our first purchase was a black and white television. We managed to get through that year living in a three-bedroom apartment.

Being from the country, we decided one year like that was enough. We found a small, three-bedroom house with a nice yard on Orchard View Lane for $16,000. Over the years, we did much painting and redecorating, but in 1989 we moved to a more spacious house that we had built.

In 1972, I began working as a part-time secretary for an insurance agent, In 1975, I changed jobs, and began working half-time as the bookkeeper for the Aerospace and Ocean Engineering Department on campus. After the children were grown, I decided to work full-time, and I took the bookkeeper's position at the conference center on campus. Glenn had left his original alfalfa-breeding job to become the soybean breeder for the university. Paula attended and graduated from Virginia Tech in mechanical engineering, and Gary graduated from Rochester Institute of Technology with an associate degree in photography.

During 1983, I believe we had one of the roughest years of our married life. My father's health was deteriorating: he was suffering from hardening of the arteries and congestive heart failure. From December 1982 until his death on May 17, 1983, I, of course, could not think of much else. It was very sad to see my father, who had always been the strong figure in the family, slowly lose his memory and his grasp on life.

A month after his death, Paula graduated from college, and two weeks later she was married to Russell Lindsay. They immediately moved to Cincinnati, Ohio, where they both had accepted engineering positions with General Electric. The next big job that needed to be done was to clean out my father's house so that it could be sold. I was not looking forward to that one bit. The task itself was bad enough, but it was further complicated by the strained relations between the siblings that had existed for years. All of us working in one house together was not my idea of the way to spend my vacation. As it turned out, things went okay, but certainly not without bitterness. I learned the meaning of the expression about "cutting the tension with a knife"!

Chapter 3

The Family Matures Well

I figured that was water over the dam, and the next item of business was to move Gary into an apartment in Rochester, where he would finish his second year at RIT. That seemed to be just fine for a month or so, until Gary informed us that he was not happy with his inconsiderate roommates and was going to move out. He found a house with five other students and somehow moved himself. I guess all parents find that when your twenty-year-old starts making his own decisions, you begin to get a few more gray hairs. He seemed to manage, and we didn't have two apartments to pay rent on for that school year after all! By the end of that year, he had wrecked his Mustang during a snowstorm—not too bad; it still worked and no one was seriously injured. He found himself a girlfriend and a summer job in New York City.

Blacksburg is a typical small college town, and I had never been to New York City. Gary went there for the first time with a friend from RIT. He walked the streets of the 'photo district,' and after two visits he felt certain he had found what he wanted with the David Langley Studio.

7

After he finished that school year, he visited a few days with us before heading for the Big Apple. His first week he stayed at the YMCA Sloane House. I didn't hear from him until the next weekend. There are all sorts of things that enter a mother's mind under such conditions, but as usual he made it again. He knew not a soul and quickly learned how to use the subway and even how to drive in the city.

He soon got an apartment in Brooklyn, and by September his lease had run out. Against Mom and Dad's wishes, he decided to quit school and rent another apartment in Brooklyn. At this time, his girlfriend also decided to quit school and get a job in the city. This meant they would be living together and sharing expenses. (Glenn and I are both Christians and had brought the children up in the church, so this was not something we agreed with, but learned to accept.) They both seemed to like their photography jobs and be quite happy.

With our children 'settled' and Glenn and I both working full-time, we were beginning to enjoy life. We could begin to feel a sense of freedom. Plus, with no college tuition bills coming every three months, the financial burden had been lifted. I really enjoyed my job, worked with some fun people and can honestly say that I don't think I could have had better working conditions anywhere else. I belonged to an evening bridge club, while Glenn and I belonged to a couples' dinner bridge group as well as a square dance club. We were both quite active in the Lutheran Church. I was the treasurer, Glenn was a council member, and we shared the job of changing the paraments (the cloths on the pulpit, altar and other parts of a church sanctuary). We also attended many of the functions held at the university, so our social calendar was full.

Chapter 4

Something Just Doesn't Seem Right

In September of 1984, Paula and Russ were relocated for four months to work in San Francisco as part of a training program for GE. For that reason, plus the National Agronomy Meetings scheduled to be in Las Vegas the week after Thanksgiving, we decided to vacation out there for a week and a half. About a week before we left, I went to my family doctor because I had been experiencing weakness in my hands. I had first noticed it when I was writing. He checked me and told me that I had probably sprained my ligaments when I carried several loads of firewood into our basement for our fireplace. That put my mind at ease.

Glenn and I left the Roanoke airport on the Wednesday morning before Thanksgiving and met Paula and Russ in San Francisco that afternoon. The balance of that day and the following four days were packed full of all the sightseeing events in the area that time allowed. My sister, Madelyn, and her husband, Beanie, had come from

Pennsylvania to join us for a couple of those days. We all had a great time. The only problems we encountered were: (1) our luggage did not arrive on the same plane we did; and (2) our Sunday flight to Las Vegas was canceled without anyone having notified us.

As it turned out, our luggage arrived the day after we got to San Francisco, and we were fortunate enough to catch a flight out Monday morning to 'Sin City.' Glenn and I had never been to a gambling town, so this was an all new experience. We had the best time! Glenn attended meetings during the day, and I went on tours planned for the spouses. Every night we went to different shows, and while we were there we fed enough slot machines to rid our pockets of $20. We left there very reluctantly on Thursday morning. The trip was wonderful, and the only problem I encountered was some difficulty writing postcards.

We settled back into our work routine the following Monday. Two weeks went by, and my hands were a bit weaker and my legs had a hint of weakness when I climbed steps. Before heading to Pennsylvania and New York for the Christmas holidays, I decided to stop in to see my family doctor to find out why the problem was getting worse. After checking me, he seemed a bit puzzled and decided to send me to a neurologist in Roanoke when I returned from our holiday vacation. I left his office and walked home (about a mile) as I usually did everyday after work.

We had a nice Christmas with both our children gathering at Glenn's folks' home. After Paula and Russ flew back to Cincinnati, Glenn and I drove Janet and Gary back to New York. When I was a child, I had lived just about 120 miles from the city, but had never had an opportunity to go there. Needless to say, it was quite an experience! We stayed that night with Janet and Gary in their one-bedroom Brooklyn apartment. We did go to dinner and a show, riding the subway from Brooklyn to Manhattan. That was our first experience—not a bad one, but one that led me to believe I would stick to small-town living.

Putting on my gloves was a very difficult chore, along with hooking my bra and carrying heavy items, but other than that I seemed to manage okay. We returned to Blacksburg, went to a New Year's Eve party, and sat around watching TV on New Year's Day. I was sitting on the floor in front of the fireplace when the phone rang. I got up to answer it, and—to my surprise—I fell backward. After that, I noticed that when I climbed the stairs, my legs did seem a bit weaker. And holding the phone was getting to be a strain on my hands.

That afternoon, Glenn and I went to the drugstore to get a large ace bandage, thinking that if I wrapped my forearm, perhaps it would give me some support and make it feel better. The next morning I went to work; writing and typing were possible, but not easy. I called my family physician, Dr. Boatwright, and told him that my problem had worsened and I would like to see the neurologist sooner than January 14, when my original appointment had been scheduled. He, being such a caring person, immediately made arrangements for me to see the specialist that afternoon.

I called Glenn on that rainy day, told him I could now see the neurologist that afternoon, and noted we would have to leave soon to make the appointment. I quickly finished a few things on my desk, then told my office-mates and supervisor that I was leaving and probably wouldn't be back until the next morning.

11

It is about a 45-minute drive from Blacksburg to Roanoke. Once Glenn had picked me up, I immediately removed the ace bandages, because they just didn't seem to help much. In the car, we ate our packed lunch, which we usually ate together each day in Glenn's office. We made our appointment on time, but as in any doctors' offices, you hurry up and wait. I was the doctor's last appointment for the day.

When I first met this doctor, I was impressed with his manner and his examination. He determined that there was a problem with the spinal column in the neck area and suggested that I go to the hospital as soon as possible for further tests. My thought was that it was something that surgery would correct, and the sooner I got it over with, the better it would be. So, Glenn and I talked it over, and we decided I would go over to the hospital as soon as I could buy a few pieces of clothing at a nearby shopping center. We then went over to the Roanoke Memorial Hospital, where I was admitted as an emergency case. Even under those conditions I did not have any trouble getting a private room, which pleased me. The room was very nice and had a private bath, which at that point, I was able to use myself.

For the next four days I was poked with many needles. I was given the myelogram, CT scan and blood tests. On Sunday, January 6, just before being released from the hospital, I was given the EMG. The doctor talked to Glenn and me after he administered the EMG. He said there was nothing from any of the tests that indicated surgery should be performed. My first question was, "Do I have MS?"

"No," the doctor replied, "that has been ruled out." He continued: "It is probably a virus of some kind, or a motor neuron disease. Just go home. I'll set up an appointment for you to come to my office in three weeks." He wanted to keep checking on it, and if things worsened, he would send me to either the University of Virginia in Charlottesville or Duke University in North Carolina.

Well, Glenn took me home, and we still didn't know what was causing my frustrating problem. I did not go back to work, having been worn out from the hospital visit. A couple of days passed, and I came down with the 24-hour flu. That seemed to weaken me even more. I could not even pick up a blanket to fold it, and my legs were showing more weakness. What a frightening experience! I was getting desperate to find out just what was happening to me. I called the Roanoke doctor, who had me run all the way up there and charged me $35 to tell me I wasn't much worse than I had been when he saw me in the hospital. I was to come back on the 28th for my next appointment. Glenn and I returned home a bit be-wildered. I was unable to work, but I was able to still do some things at home. A few days went by and things seemed to worsen.

It finally just got to the point that I wanted some answers. I called the neurologist in Roanoke to ask him to please send me somewhere for more tests. By January 16, I had been admitted to UVA, about a three-hour drive from our home. Glenn, again leaving his work behind, drove me to Charlottesville, picking up my records from the Roanoke doctor on the way. We arrived at 7:30 that Wednesday evening. I assumed that testing would begin in the morning. Wrong! They began immediately, with two female doctors giving me their own individual exams. The evening ended at 10:30 with a spinal tap.

The UVA research hospital is large, but the buildings are very old. Private rooms are almost unheard of. I guess I was lucky to be in a semi-private room, with a commode and sink. I was still able to manage the bathroom chores myself, but holding the hairdryer was not something I could do. Opening a milk carton was difficult, showering was difficult and walking was not too hard, but climbing steps was becoming more of an effort.

The doctor who performed the spinal tap right in my bed failed to tell me that I was to lie flat for the next four hours. Soon after the doctors finished working on me, a nurse came to "tuck me in" for the night. When I got up to go to the bathroom, the nurse noticed the remains of the supplies used for the spinal tap by my bed and informed me I was not to be standing up. I was quite annoyed over the fact that since the doctor had said nothing to that effect, I could have had a very bad headache; but, afraid to move, I lay perfectly still till 2:00 a. m. Fortunately, I did not develop any side effects.

I really don't think I had much more than two hours' sleep that night. The atmosphere for sleeping was not like going to a Hilton! The next morning came, and many doctors came by my bedside, all doing the same types of tests. They checked my reflexes, fingers to nose, nose to toes, standing on one foot. They asked me many questions. I even had the head of neurology come by with about six of his students. They congregated in the hall before seeing me and after seeing me. I, being naive about the whole thing, still was not aware of all the interest in me. I guess I just assumed everyone in that hospital got that same type of attention. One of the doctors asked me if I had any idea what might be wrong or some of the consequences I might have to face. I replied, "No, but it has been a question that I was afraid to ask."

He asked me then to walk down the hall with him to a place where we would have some privacy. Sure that we would not be overheard, he told me that, while it had not been fully determined, signs were pointing toward motor neuron disease. He added that eventually I would probably need help, possibly even to the point of making some changes in the home to accommodate a wheelchair. All I thought of was Glenn and how he was going to do it. I guess I accepted that in a sense, but I wasn't to that point yet, so I wanted to put the prospects out of my mind.

I returned to my room, where soon a few more doctors came by to talk with me. Then it was suggested that I might have Amyotrophic Lateral Sclerosis. That could not definitely be determined until I had the EMG run. The next step was to go to a room where they would do the final test. They first had me put my arms and legs in very warm water. Then they laid me on the table and inserted a type of needle in my legs, arms and hand muscles. The needle was connected to a machine that showed nerve impulse readings on a screen that looked much like a computer screen.

After that was completed, they went on to an even more painful test done with electrodes placed on certain arm and leg muscles. They would first do one leg, putting a small amount of current through the first time, working the current up to a body-jolting shock on the fourth shot. This continued until each leg and arm had a sample of the shock treatment. These results also showed on the screen, and the two doctors who administered the test watched intently as the electricity showed just what they had thought it would—I had ALS.

I kept asking, "Just what is it?"

The reply was: a motor neuron disease called "Amyotrophic Lateral Sclerosis," a disease that attacks only the motor nerves. I knew then that it was serious, but not exactly how serious. They called an orderly to take me back to my room. After returning, I saw a familiar face in the hall. I started a conversation with her and found she was from Blacksburg. Her husband had been ill for at least a year and was on disability from Virginia Tech. She then wondered why I was there. I told her, and she informed me that ALS was Lou Gehrig's Disease.

That is when it hit me. I didn't have long to live! Then my mind started reviewing the events of the past day and a half. The one doctor had been paged while examining me. When she used my phone to check in, she said she could not leave until she finished because she was working on an acute case. And when the head neur-ologist had showed his class the lack of reflexes in my arms and the unusual reflexes in my legs, he informed them that there was already weakness in the left side of my throat.

Thoughts began to fill my mind to the point that sleeping was impossible. The next morning, a doctor who was managing my records told me that I would be given a prescription to take to an occupational therapist in Roanoke and to a physical therapist in Blacksburg. He also told me I would be released that day because there was no need for me to stay any longer. I then told him I was going to 'fight it,' and he sarcastically replied, "Aren't we all?"

Chapter 5

Happy Birthday!

I called Glenn, broke the news to him and told him I would be released by noon. He drove up from Blacksburg, crying most all the way. He broke down again as soon as he hit my room door, which was filled with balloons sent to me by my officemates for my 43rd birthday. For some reason, I kept a stiff upper lip. I told Glenn we would have to take each day at a time, and I would try to fight it the best way I could. Glenn waited while I had one more test run before being released. That was a breathing test, which took about fifteen minutes. I was put in two different booths for two different tests.

I returned to my room, and two or three doctors came to meet with Glenn and me to give us the official diagnosis and a 'brief' synopsis of the disease. They then said it was what the doctor in Roanoke suspected, ALS. They added that there was no approved medication, but that a drug—Thyrotropin Releasing Hormone (TRH)—had been experimented with over the past two years, with some good results. There were a few places in the United States working with it, but only the University of Wisconsin would have an opening. This seemed pretty exciting to me,

17

so I told the neurologist in charge that I wanted to try it. He then said he would make the arrangements, suggesting that perhaps as early as February 1, I could be in Wisconsin. He explained that since he would be turning me back over to the office in Roanoke, he would call my neurologist there, since it would be closer to home.

After signing many release forms and packing my clothes, Glenn and I walked out of the hospital, with much sadness in our hearts along with a spark of hope.

Chapter 6

Searching for Answers

When Glenn and I arrived in Blacksburg, it was already cold and dark. We stopped at the drugstore to have a sleeping pill prescription filled. As we waited, I gazed over the many items on display, that people used to help them walk. I jokingly mentioned to Glenn that I would soon be getting one of those. He just said, "That won't be for a while."

I remember thinking to myself that I was sure it wouldn't, because I wasn't going to let that happen. I planned to fight it! We then drove home where we found our dear neighbor, Mary Jenkins, making up our bed. She knew I was unable to do that, and Glenn had all he could do just to get to work and run me all around. She immediately wanted to know what the results of the tests had been. I told her, and said things would not get better. She was almost speechless and hurried to finish her job so she could exit as fast as she could. She later told me she went home and asked her husband, Dave, what Lou Gehrig's disease was. She had heard of it, but didn't know much about it.

The next thing we knew, the phone was ringing. Our daughter had called to wish me a "Happy Birthday." I had not told the children that I had gone for more tests, because I didn't want to worry them unnecessarily. I then told her the results and told her about the drug that was being administered in Wisconsin, knowing that would be my only hope. Soon Gary called and I had to break the news to him. They were both in a state of shock, but tried hard to put the inevitable out of their minds.

The next day Glenn wanted me to go to the shopping mall with him to look for a speaker telephone that I would be able to use without holding a receiver, which was very tiring for my weak hands. I remember standing around the store for about ten minutes, and then I had to go out and sit on a bench while Glenn made the purchase. My legs were beginning to tire easily.

After we got the phone hooked up and read all the instructions, we decided to call Madelyn and Beanie and Glenn's parents. None of them wanted to believe what we were saying. They had never heard of the disease and certainly could not believe that my life would be cut short. It just couldn't be true. Something like this always seems to happen to other people, how could this happen to us? The next day many of my friends began to call. By the next week the news had gotten around town. The food, flowers and cards began pouring in.

Between answering the door and the phone, Glenn didn't get much else done. He did go to the office when he could, but he said he couldn't get anything done because all he could think about was me. It was like Grand Central Station around the house. My neighbor looks back on it now and says it reminded her of a funeral home. So many people just couldn't believe it.

I wanted to do something, but didn't know what to do. Everyone's thoughtfulness was greatly appreciated. I told Glenn I was glad to see so many flowers before my funeral. I had never received many flower arrangements during my lifetime, but I surely made up for it during the months that followed. Days seemed to be filled with activity, but the nights seemed long. Before going to bed, I took a very mild sleeping pill that lasted exactly four hours, and then my eyes would pop open and many thoughts would wander through my mind. With only four hours' sleep each night, I felt like I was walking around in a fog.

I had been told to call the neurologist in Roanoke the week after arriving home from Charlottesville to see just when I would be going to the University of Wisconsin. Well, to begin with, the Roanoke doctor had never heard from the doctor at UVA, so he said he would call him and get back with me. I was quite hopeful at this point that I would be flying to Wisconsin soon. Patiently, I waited to hear from the Roanoke doctor. When I got his call, I just couldn't believe what I was hearing. He told me that the people at UVA had done nothing about calling Wisconsin and that he certainly saw no reason for my going out there. He had read nothing to indicate that TRH was of much benefit, and besides, he said, "You could go into remission anytime."

Being very bitter and disappointed with his reaction, I asked him what he would do if he were in my shoes? He then very reluctantly said he would talk with the University of Wisconsin. The next phone call came from his secretary telling me that they could not reach the University of Wisconsin Neurology Department. Then she gave me the number to call them myself.

Now, when I look back on the months that followed, it makes my head spin! I finally got in contact with Dr. Ben

Brooks' office. He was the doctor in charge of the TRH experiments. His staff told me to have my records sent immediately, which I did. They had indicated to me that, once my records were received, they would review them and then would call me when and if they would be using me. I guess when I was talking with the secretaries out there, I heard what I had wanted to hear! I knew that I would be called, and I was sitting on pins and needles just waiting for that phone call.

After Gary heard the news, he began asking his co-workers about ALS. One of them knew a woman who was going to a doctor in New York, who was supposed to be the best for anyone with ALS. Well, I immediately made an appointment and had my records forwarded. We were about to buy our plane tickets, when Gary checked things out more thoroughly and found that this doctor had nothing more to offer than the doctors at UVA— occupational and physical therapy. That high passed rather quickly.

When the next weekend rolled around, Paula and Russ drove from Cincinnati and Gary flew down from New York. It certainly was not one of our happiest family gatherings! The feelings of a lump in your throat and lead in your stomach seemed to always be there. I could still walk and do some things with my hands at this point, but to do daily chores was not possible. Paula did the laundry, made the meals and ran the vacuum before returning home that Sunday afternoon. Gary stayed until Thursday and then returned to New York to terminate his job and to try to sublet his apartment so he could return home to help his father take care of me. Glenn and I certainly did not want to uproot him and take him from his career, but being a very sensitive and caring person he wanted to do it.

Glenn was planning to continue going to work, coming home at lunch to check on me. Visitors and food were still plentiful at this point, and we were managing quite well under the circumstances. After returning to New York, Gary immediately got on the phone, called his grandparents, my sister and Paula and lined up someone to come for a week at a time so someone would be with me until he could move back home. In the meantime, so many of our friends wanted to help out in any way they could. Our neighbor, Mary, and her eight-month-old daughter, Amy, visited daily and helped do anything they could. Another dear friend drove me to Roanoke to the Rehabilitation Center for my appointment with the occupational therapist.

After spending about an hour with the therapist, it was obvious to me that she had not dealt with many ALS patients. I came away with a sponge glove for bathing, which when made wet was too heavy for my weak muscles to pick up. She wanted me to buy utensils for arthritic hands, but I refused that offer, knowing they were also too heavy. She thought I could use a long stick with pincers to help me pick things up from the floor, but that, too, was of no help to me. She did insist that I take a no-slide sheet to put under my plate when eating. I took it only to put it away, since my hands were too weak to make even my plate slide. I also came away from there a bit more morbid.

She gave me a list of things I would need and said to call the telephone number she gave me for someone to deliver whatever was needed. On the list was a raised commode seat. It was becoming more and more difficult for me to get up from a chair, and this would make going to the bathroom a little easier for me. Also on that list were bars for alongside the commode, a shower bench and a wheelchair with a mouth stick and arm straps.

When I returned home and showed Glenn just what I was going to need, he began to cry. What really bothered me was knowing what I could expect to come even after the wheelchair: the respirator to help my breathing and the horrible suffering for me and the family. The next day I ordered the high toilet seat and the shower bench. I didn't feel I was quite ready for that wheelchair yet.

A few days passed, and Glenn took me out to the local hospital to see a physical therapist. I really did not want to go. The occupational therapist at UVA had led me to believe that a physical therapist was of little use with this disease. To my surprise, I was greeted by Irmtraut Hartenstein, a friend from our church, who had been assigned to my case. She tried to explain the disease to Glenn and me, which had never been done in detail before. She told us she had worked with several ALS patients and some lived for many years after being diagnosed. She said to try anything that would be offered, even if it meant traveling to Wisconsin to get it, because you never know when a breakthrough will come.

As she was talking to us and putting us at ease (as much as one can be under the circumstances), she was showing us various exercises that I should do daily. She then told us to call her anytime, and rather than our coming by the hospital each week she would be stopping by our house to check on me. As we left, Glenn and I both felt that Irmtraut was the most informative and concerned person in the medical profession with whom we had talked since we had been told I had the dreaded disease.

My sister, Madelyn, came to stay with Glenn and me for two weeks. She had done nothing but take care of someone since she and Beanie were married in 1965. First, she helped my mother during her very painful and long fight with cancer till she passed away in 1969. Then she was there for my father through his many years of loneliness and failing health. When he passed away, she was ready to enjoy her life and hoped to do some traveling without the worry of something happening at home. Little did she dream she would have to help care for her sister, who everyone thought was strong, healthy and active! From the time I first told her about my illness, she had been researching and reading anything she could get her hands on. Her interests in vitamins had begun several years prior to this, when she started drinking a high-protein mix for a nervous problem she was experiencing. So, since she had seen some improvement, she started me on the same drink and changed my diet. I was eating fish, chicken, fresh fruits and vegetables, no red meat or preserved fruits or vegetables. This was continued faithfully for three months.

While she was with us, I could walk out to the car, but I didn't go into stores because my legs would tire easily. Steps were already impossible without assistance. Glenn did anything he could to make things easier for me, and the next thing to do was to build a ramp so I could avoid the two small steps we had at the back of the house.

By the time we took Madelyn to the airport to fly back to Pennsylvania, Paula had arrived. She took personal leave from her job to spend the week with me. She was able to take me for rides in the car. I could walk on level surfaces, but I needed to be pulled up when I was in a sitting position. After we took Paula back to the airport, Glenn's parents arrived so they could take their turn at caring for me. His mother, Evelyn, was afraid there wouldn't be enough to keep her busy once she got here, but it didn't take her long to find out that there was plenty to do, with barely enough hours in a day! Pop kept busy by painting the ramp, pruning trees and doing some grocery shopping.

I was still receiving many phone calls and lots of company. At times I could hear the low voices in another room, obviously talking about my grave condition! Anyway, one of my visitors was my supervisor from work. He came to bring my termination papers by for me to sign. While visiting, he told me of a friend of his who was thought to have ALS, but after checking with another doctor had found that he was low on Vitamin B12. Well, you guessed it! I immediately called my family doctor, Dr. Boatwright. He, probably feeling my frustration, said if I wanted to try the B12 shots, he'd be glad to give them to me. Glenn took me to the office, where the nurse was going to show him how to administer the shots so he could give them to me twice a week.

While I was walking into the office, I tripped over a small step and took my first fall. Once that happens, it completely destroys your confidence. This just about ended my walking anywhere without assistance by my side. Glenn continued giving me the shots for the next couple of months. I remembered my mother telling me that she would go for a Vitamin B12 shot every once in a while, and it would give her a burst of energy. Well, I never experienced any such thing. In fact, when there was no improvement with this treatment, I decided I was not low on B12!

I stayed in the house while Glenn went out to bid his parents good-bye. He hated to see them go, and just thinking about me made him break down. I later learned that his parents shed tears over half the way home. There is some sick feeling that seems to never go away when something like this strikes someone you care for.

By the beginning of March, Gary and his girlfriend, Janet DiFabio, had quit their jobs and moved much of their furniture into his grandparents' already overcrowded house. They arrived about five o'clock on that Tuesday afternoon. Driving a VW Rabbit for eight hours had left them a bit weary, but since they were young, that didn't stop them from unloading their packed car. They moved everything into our basement, where they would have their own bedroom and the family room, which soon was turned into a photography studio. The TV was downstairs along with a fireplace.

By this time the only way for me to get downstairs was if Glenn or Gary carried me. I didn't like them to do that— I had a tremendous fear of falling—so Glenn bought me a small color TV with remote controls for our bedroom. For this reason, many hours of my day were spent in the bedroom. I was never alone for very long; but if for some reason no one was in the house, I would stay on the bed with the remote control and telephone. I was still able to push the buttons. Because of my fear of falling, I never walked unless someone was around.

During January and February I made frequent calls to the University of Wisconsin (UW), but to no avail. We had neighbors, Lisa and Brock Metcalf, a sweet couple who were both doing graduate work at Virginia Tech. They, too, wanted to help. It happened that Lisa's father was a lawyer in Washington for the American Medical Association. Lisa told him about my situation, and he tried to get me into the Thyrotropin Releasing Hormone (TRH) testing program. He tried in every way possible, but that, too, turned out to be fruitless. Another friend, with whom I had worked three years prior to this time, called and told me that a cousin of hers was married to an ophthalmologist who worked at UW, and she was going to talk with him and see what he could do. He was also kind enough to go to Dr. Brooks' office to see how he could help get me into the program. And still another friend from the church who had some connections out there also had someone put a word in for me, but I was never called.

Finally, Gary had had enough of the waiting game. Because I was still hopeful that I would be called, he put a call through to Dr. Brooks, who was kind enough to return the call and tell Gary he hoped to start working on getting TRH approved by the FDA. He suggested it would probably be just as easy on me to wait for that as to go to Wisconsin. That seemed to give me even greater hope!

Since the date of April 1 was mentioned in Gary's conversation with Dr. Brooks, I again thinking what I wanted to think was hoping by that date my local physician would be able to administer the drug. Well, that date came and went, and I again started bugging the UW office. Always, I was given the tender loving care conversation. Finally, I realized this was all pretty much false hope that I was dealing with.

Chapter 7

Juice and Vitamins

When Gary came home to care for me, he was certain somehow I just had to get better. He and Janet were going to much trouble to fix all the right kinds of food for me. I never had red meat, anything made with white flour or white sugar. I was sure that perhaps a good diet could at least stop the disease from progressing, but it seemed as each week went by I was able to do a little less.

Gary shopped for many of my foods at the health food store in town. One day, he struck up a conversation with the manager and told him about my terminal illness. Eager to help, the manager suggested that carrot juice might help cure my ailment. The theory was it would clean my system. He also suggested a coffee enema. Being desperate, I went along with the carrot juice, but not the enema. To me, this seemed to be a sure cure. After hearing of several success stories, I knew it could work for me if I just could stick to it. Since we had no juicer, we spent more than $200 on one so that I could have fresh juice daily. We went through approximately 25 pounds of carrots a week. The big glass of carrot juice being given to me every three hours is not something I look back on with delight!

With this and my weekly vitamin regimen, plus the intake of new vitamins from my sister, I thought surely improvement would follow. I'm not sure just how many vitamins I was taking, but by April it was a lot, from primrose oil to calcium and thyroid pills. Paula, being so far away and unable to do as much as she wished she could, was also trying every avenue to find something to help my deteriorating condition. She found a chiro-practor and nutrition specialist who had had success working with multiple sclerosis patients, so she went to talk with him. He was willing to give her a "supply" of vitamins and supplements, the cost of which amounted to more than $250, which she immediately sent to me. She then made an appointment for me to see him the Friday before Memorial Day.

I was still doing daily exercises with assistance, with Irmtraut taking time from her busy schedule to check on me periodically. In March she had talked with my family physician about trying an electrical stimulator, which was battery controlled. This was something that had not been tried on an ALS patient before, at least in this area. Well, Dr. Boatwright again gave his approval. Irmtraut brought over the "little black box," which I was eager to try. I thought I would get renewed strength. She attached it to my belt while I had the electrodes taped to the muscles on my legs or arms. This would give me a shock every half second or so. I did this every morning, doing different sets of muscles for about eight minutes each. It took about an hour and a half, with either Gary or Janet changing the electrodes every ten minutes.

The idea was that the shock would stimulate the nerve to that muscle and possibly prevent muscle atrophy. The equipment cost $100 a month to rent. Irmtraut really didn't know how it would work in my situation, but she was willing to try anything to allow me to walk longer. I continued the exercises through May. She even rigged the equipment up so I could wear it on my legs when I walked, with a switch in one shoe that would alternate the current to my legs as I went.

By the middle of May, I had taken my third fall. It frightened me so that I walked only with either Gary or Glenn holding me under my arms. When I told Irmtraut about it, she immediately brought a walker for me to try. It had four wheels and armrests with handles for my hands. At this point my arms and hands were too weak to lift a regular walker, but I was able to push this one. It was a great help, because I could at least get to the bathroom and lean on that while someone pulled my slacks and underwear off in order for me to go to the toilet.

The morning I fell, Glenn was getting ready to go on a business trip. Starting to cry, I told him I'd probably never walk again. He, too, felt bad, but tried to console me. Each time I fell my knees would take the brunt of the fall, and it would take a couple of weeks for them to get their strength back, what little there was! That morning, Glenn left with tear-filled eyes.

A few months earlier, a friend from the church had offered me her late husband's wheelchair. It was practically new, and she insisted she would be delighted for us to use it. Glenn picked it up one Sunday morning, and I did use it to go outside or to the mall occasionally. I also went to church until I could no longer walk from the wheelchair into the pew. I got my taste of just how a handicapped person feels. Because you are in a wheel-chair, people are at a loss for words, and they have pity written all over their faces. That, I know, wasn't my problem, but I just hated going into crowds, especially in our hometown of Blacksburg.

Nelda Buss

Chapter 8

Anyone Need a Rest Stop?

Memorial Day, 1985, was fast approaching, and I was still on the diet, drinking carrot juice and taking about fourteen pills a day. By this time, carrot juice had been part of my daily intake for about two months, and I was beginning to notice that I was feeling dizzy or lightheaded after drinking it each time. I told Gary this, but he did not want to believe it, because he thought this was the one thing that was going to get me better. When he talked with his good buddy at the health food store, he was told that it probably was just the way you might feel before you would begin to feel better!

Walking was difficult even with the walker. I could get to the bathroom and bedroom with it, but I tried not to make any more trips than necessary. I was looking forward to making the trip to Cincinnati to see Paula. It was going to be my first long trip in the car since I had begun my fight. We decided to take a bedpan, changing pad, paper bag and Kleenex along with my wheelchair and walker. That meant our trunk was filled even though we took as little luggage as possible. Glenn had been fighting a sore throat for three

33

days prior to leaving, but he said he guessed he would be okay and we could go anyway. So, off we went.

About four hours after we started, we stopped at a rest stop on the West Virginia Turnpike. I needed a man to help me in and out of the car and wheelchair. Janet was always good to help me, but she did not want to take me to the bathroom without a male for fear that I might fall. Even though public places may have facilities for the handicapped, they are often not very convenient to use. I'm sure most women would not object to a man appearing in the ladies room under the circumstances, but I would not do that. So, after we ate our packed lunch (I had a chicken sandwich, made with health food bread, celery and grapes.), which I needed assistance with, we drove our car to a far corner of the parking lot and set up our own latrine! Gary held me up off of the car seat while Janet laid down the changing pad and Glenn pulled down my pants and slid the bedpan beneath me. When I was finished, they threw the Kleenex, used for toilet paper, in a paper bag that went into the garbage, and the urine was discarded in the grass in the pet area! Everyone else then used the restrooms, and we were on our way again.

When we arrived at Paula and Russ' apartment, they took me in on the wheelchair. They then lifted me up from the chair so I could walk with the walker. I walked maybe ten steps to the bathroom, and then about that many to the dining room table. It did not go easy. In fact, I hated the thought of having to get up to walk anywhere, because it was such a chore. Paula had fixed a nice meal for all of us, even going to the trouble to fix fresh fruits and vegetables for me. At bedtime, Gary picked me up and carried me upstairs. When he was in high school he was a wrestler and lifted weights. At the time I didn't care for it, fearing all the time that he might get hurt. He did get his nose broken in practice one day and that tended to stifle his enthusiasm for wrestling. But now that those days had passed, I was very glad for the muscles he had developed.

The next morning, I walked with the walker, with Glenn by my side, to the bathroom. I got seated on the toilet where Glenn gave me a sponge bath. This was something we started after I could no longer stand in the shower. After Glenn washed me, brushed my teeth and got me dressed, Gary carried me back downstairs for breakfast. I could still eat myself, but I had to use plastic knives and forks, because regular silverware was too heavy for me to handle. After breakfast they loaded me back up in the car, and we followed Paula's instructions to the chiropractor's office.

This was really something I was looking forward to; it was another spark of hope. Glenn took me into the office where we met the doctor, who asked me many questions. We discussed the reaction I was having to the carrot juice, which sounded to him like an allergic reaction. Well, that ended the carrot juice therapy! He then went over the vast list of vitamins that I had been consuming for three or four weeks. The whole mess was making me feel like I had an upset stomach most of the time, and my muscle weakness was worsening. He suggested that I go back to the other vitamins I had been taking before I started his program and add the ones he had prescribed gradually. His partner met me and gave me an "adjustment," after which I returned to the main part of the office, where I answered a questionnaire. (Glenn, of course, filled in the answers for me, since I could no longer write.) This would determine what flower and herb oils would be put into a potion that could help my various moods. Finally, the chiropractor suggested that I have my records forwarded to him, on the premise that I could have been misdiagnosed. We then left his office with the flower oils, a bottle of homeopathic drops and more than $75 less in our checking account after paying for the medicines and office call.

The next day, Paula and Russ took all of us to the Cincinnati Zoo. We had a nice day, and it was a pleasant change for me. That evening we played Trivial Pursuit until 11:30 and then went to bed. Sunday morning both Glenn I awoke with a sore throat. His was a little worse, and mine was just beginning. We left for home after breakfast. On the way I sucked on zinc tablets. I had heard that they were the miracle cure for a sore throat. The next day was Memorial Day, and neither Glenn nor I felt well. In fact, Glenn felt so bad that he went to the doctor that afternoon. Both he and I had a fever. The doctor prescribed an antibiotic for both of us, having determined we had a bacterial infection. By the next evening we both had developed a cough that caused us to get very little sleep for the following few days.

Chapter 9

Cheer Up!
Things Could Be Worse

Through all of this, I was still able to walk with the walker, but a week later I found both my arms and legs becoming weaker. And by the time the next week had passed, I found myself completely motionless from my neck down. Then reality began to set in, and everyone who knew me was probably thinking the same thing as I: "What will be next and when?" Even though my fever and my cough had subsided, my throat just did not seem quite right. In fact, I gagged on some of the vitamin pills.

At that point I decided, "I don't need these pills or the troublesome diet." I figured if I were going to get better from that, I wouldn't be in the shape I was in now. Boy, did Janet's spaghetti ever taste good! I called Dr. Boatwright about my throat. He, being the Good Samaritan that he is, came to the house to check on me. I was in the wheelchair when he arrived. I told him I was sorry I couldn't walk to the door or shake his hand. He wittily replied, "I know, but you can still use that mouth of yours!"

That's something for which I am thankful to this day. The doctor said I had taken too many antibiotics, and that had caused a yeast infection in my throat. I quit taking the antibiotics, and within a couple of weeks' time, my throat was feeling better. By then, though, my diaphragm had weakened, which made my coughing and nose-blowing much weaker. And I noticed that when Glenn or Gary would pick me up under my arms, my voice would not come out. I thought it might be a result of my inactivity, but I later found out differently.

Everything else seemed to be in fine working order. I still had my monthly periods and had regular bladder and bowel activity. I had always been a very private person, but anyone who is stricken with ALS might as well decide that privacy will have to go, at least when both the arms and legs are affected. Between Glenn, Gary and Janet my needs were well taken care of; not always with relish, but they got done. The problems that came with being paralyzed were not something that anyone but a paraplegic could ever imagine. The fear of falling was something that I could not overcome. When Glenn put me on the bed, he had to make sure I was sitting in just the right position. Otherwise, I would fall backward, with no way of breaking my fall. For this reason I hated the thoughts of getting my showers. Glenn would put me on the shower bench, which had no side rails, and I was fearful of every move till I was put back into the wheelchair. No matter how much I was reassured that I would be fine, it did not make me feel secure.

Taking me to the bathroom was another situation that had to be dealt with. Either Gary or Glenn had to be present when I went to the bathroom. They would pick me up, while someone else, usually Janet, pulled my elastic-waist slacks and underwear down. In order to wipe me, they had to hold my knees apart with their knee and hand. I had no control of my legs at all.

Right after I became unable to move anything, sleeping became very difficult. Poor Glenn had to move me about every two hours. Pressure on different spots of my body seemed unbearable at times. I got a sheepskin to put in the bed to help prevent bedsores. Fortunately, I never had any.

In June, soon after I became totally helpless, Madelyn and Beanie came for a week in order to give Gary and Janet a little vacation. While they were here, we decided that since sleeping was becoming a very uncomfortable time for me and my struggle was disturbing Glenn throughout the night, perhaps I could sleep in a reclining chair. Also, my feet had begun to swell soon after I was confined to the wheelchair. They were so big that I was no longer able to wear shoes. A recliner would let me keep my feet elevated and thus reduce the swelling.

So, Glenn loaded me up in the car, and the four of us were off to visit furniture stores. Another fear I had was being put in and out of the car, so the less it had to be done the better I liked it. At every store I would stay in the car and wait while they surveyed the inventory. By the end of the afternoon, they had purchased a recliner.

As time went on, it seemed that trying to stay in one position at night was becoming almost impossible. One night, when Glenn was out of town, Gary was sleeping on the floor in his sleeping bag outside my bedroom door so he could hear me when I called. He decided to try putting me in a large tire inner tube to reduce the pressure on my tailbone. This seemed comfortable at first, but the longer

I lay in it, the more my back hurt, so that tactic was discarded.

The next attempt to help everyone get more sleep was my trying to sleep in the recliner. Someone would sleep on the couch so they could hear me when my body needed to be moved. Well, one night of that and we knew that wasn't the answer!

Then, a friend gave us a large piece of foam to put on my side of the bed. It resembled an egg carton, and her husband had used it while recuperating in the hospital from a heart attack. Well, that also tended to bother my back, and it made turning me even more difficult because I would stick to it. If I were just on the plain mattress, my body would slide more easily for the person turning me. We finally came up with putting foam under each hip and one shoulder, plus two pillows under my knees. I had adjusted to staying on my back the whole night, but after my knees had been in one position for two hours, the pain was almost unbearable. Eventually, we dis-covered if my legs were not exercised during the day, my knees would not bother me at night. At this point, sleep seemed to be more important than my leg exercises. Irmtraut still came by periodically, and she told us that someone should be exercising my limbs daily so my joints would not freeze. That part of the day was not one that I enjoyed. The pain in my joints when they were moved was very uncomfortable. It felt like the joint was dry, and the bones were rubbing together. At this point, I figured I would not be using my legs anymore anyway, and I could put up with bent legs.

Glenn and I had a very good relationship, and as in all marriages, sexual activities were a common practice. The saddest time for me when my muscles began to fail dramatically was when I wanted to make love but was unable to do anything but lie there. I had always been very susceptible to bladder infections, so cleanliness was a must. That meant besides having to undress me and do all the work, he had to get me up, take me to the bathroom and wash me. Needless to say, making love isn't much fun when one person has to do it all! In the beginning, I would often end up crying after it was all over, because I felt so sorry for Glenn. He was doing everything for me, and I was unable to give anything in return. It finally got to the point where my joints and even my skin seemed to hurt if any pressure at all was placed on them/it, so sex became a thing of the past.

Generally speaking, everyone accepted all of the changes very well. Gary, Janet and Glenn kept a good sense of humor, and I always tried to stay in good spirits. I took one day at a time and tried not to even think of what was to happen eventually. My visitors were one major asset for my coping with my disease. Dorothy Wiss, a very wonderful person in our church, had begun scheduling visitors daily a few months after I was diagnosed. She realized that I could no longer do much to entertain myself, certainly nothing like needlepoint, as I had been accustomed to doing. The afternoon visitors surely did help the time go by more quickly for me. Every afternoon would be different, depending on the company I had. I always enjoyed the conversations and kept up with all of the town gossip. Many people would ask me about different happenings about Blacksburg, because they figured if anyone would know, I would!

Dorothy scheduled someone to come at 2:00 to stay an hour or two. Sometimes other people would stop in, too. One day I had a total of 15 visitors. At least I didn't have much time to think about myself and get depressed. When someone came, I always insisted that either Gary or Glenn put me in the lounge chair and put the wheel-chair in the

41

bedroom, so no one would see it. I never wanted to appear sick, so Janet always fixed my hair and make-up before anyone came. Gary asked me one day if he should put some needlepoint down by the chair so no one would think there was anything wrong with me!

One of the most memorable visits was from the Lutheran student pastor and his three-year-old daughter. She knew I worked on the computer with a stick, but because I was sitting in the lounge chair motionless, she asked me where my stick was? I explained to her that it was on the table in a cup beside the computer. She glanced over at the table and then to me, then asked, "How do you get over there?"

I explained to her that Gary lifted me into the wheelchair and pushed me over there. She stood and stared at me for a minute with her big brown eyes and inquisitive look, then asked, "How do you pee-pee?"

I told her the procedure used for that operation. I couldn't help thinking to myself how intelligent she was for her age and how honest children are. I'm sure many people wondered that very same thing, but were much too embarrassed to ask.

In the mornings after my exercises, I often worked at the table with the computer, either putting data in for Glenn or writing letters. I could not do that more than an hour or two at a time, because my bottom would get sore from sitting in one position. Oftentimes someone would have to change my position during that time. It felt like the bones were protruding through the skin. I finally ordered a wheelchair cushion and sheepskin cover to help absorb the pressure. This helped some, but still two hours was the limit for sitting in one place.

During the summer months, someone would take me outside in the wheelchair to enjoy the weather. Often Gary would "drive" very fast just to hear me fuss at him! Being in the wheelchair anywhere but on the level was frightening for me. If we were going down any incline, I always insisted on having the chair tipped back. My fear of falling forward was one that truly no one could understand until he or she had been in that situation.

I loved the outdoors, and often while I sat and watched all the activities going on around me, such as mowing the lawn, pulling weeds, hanging wash or washing the car, I would get this sick feeling in my gut. It seemed to me that this disease was such a waste to any human who ever contracted it. When the disease strikes all four limbs, as it had mine, then whatever one has done before must be done for her.

One day, Glenn took me out to sit by the blueberry patch while he picked berries. When an ant crawled between my toes and starting biting me, I had to yell for Glenn to come. There was no way I could move to get rid of the thing. Many times my nose would go unscratched or my eye unrubbed. I had to lose all my modesty. I must say, I don't think many young people would do what Gary and Janet did. I certainly never dreamed that my son would ever have to dress and undress me or wipe me after I went to the bathroom. I had always been a very private person, but you might as well forget about privacy in this situation because someone is with you no matter what you do.

Never, in a million years, did I think I would be an invalid and burden my husband with caring for me. He was wonderful, always patient and willing to do anything to make me comfortable. He tried anything to make me happy. We had always joked a lot between us, and I have often said if we had really thought about our situation much it could have been right depressing, but we never dwelt on that. We felt lucky I could still talk and that we still had each other. Glenn would always tape the Johnny Carson show, and we would watch that each evening. He was such a good comedian, and he left us laughing during many of his shows.

Chapter 10

Political Action Committee of One

When I finally accepted the fact that the medical profession really had nothing to offer any ALS patient I began writing letters on the computer. At least I had my mind, so I figured I would put it to good use and see what I could do to change the situation. My first letters went to President Ronald Reagan and my congressman and senators to encourage them to hasten the FDA's approval of Thyrotropin Releasing Hormone. The responses that I received were disheartening. I found that the manufacturers of TRH had not yet submitted an application for FDA approval. And experimental use of TRH in treating Lou Gehrig's Disease had been restricted, due to the limited availability of the drug from manufacturers. Once application for approval is received, the review process generally takes a minimum of 30 months.

Senator Paul Trible did more than one would expect from a person in such a demanding job. On my behalf, he wrote not only to the FDA, but to the National Institutes of Health. Because of his concern, I was sent a very informative pamphlet about the disease, more than anyone had told me at this point. NIH stated in their letter that TRH was difficult to produce and that it did not appear to halt the continual loss of motor nerve cells that marks the disease. In addition to TRH, the drug, cyclosporine, was being tested on ALS patients, and I learned if I were interested in being considered for this trial I should have my physician contact Dr. Stanley Appel in Houston, Texas.

My next step was to write a letter to Dr. Boatwright and enclose the information I had received from Senator Trible. Dr. Boatwright got on the phone to Texas only to hear that that research study was "full up." There was no possibility that I could be a guinea pig in that program. Dr. Boatwright even looked into the possibility of getting cyclosporine and administering it himself, but that, too, was not something that would be allowed. My bubble was burst again!

Incidentally, I never heard from the President's office. I guess he was too busy recuperating from his colon cancer surgery.

I didn't stop there. My next project was to follow a lead on a German doctor. An osteopathic doctor in my hometown in Pennsylvania had gone to a seminar during which a Dr. Hans Nieper had given a very impressive speech pertaining to research he was doing in a German hospital with nerve disease patients. My sister heard about this man and acquired an address to which I could write for more information. This again popped my bubble. I received a large packet of material containing many testimonies of different patients he had treated, most of them for muscular dystrophy. Much of his treatment seemed to be through diet, which, of course, I had had my fill of!

I did show the information to Irmtraut, and since she was born in Germany and she was going back there for her summer vacation, she decided to investigate it further. Still, we learned little except that he had worked with some ALS patients. None had improved, but some were in remission. I'm not so sure that his treatment is what caused them to be in remission; often one with ALS can be in remission and for what reason no one knows.

Chapter 11

The Healers 1

The next thing that Madelyn told me about was a healer who healed every Thursday in a Baltimore church. She said Floyd Ike, a man who belonged to her church and had ALS, had gone to Olga Worral, the healer, and was completely healed. She got the address of Mrs. Worral and suggested I write to her. I was certainly not very optimistic about such a thing, but I figured it certainly wouldn't hurt anything. I soon received a reply, only to find out that Olga Worral had passed away about the same time I was diagnosed. I was to be put on the prayer list at the Methodist church in Baltimore, where healing services continued even after Olga's death. Healing was done every Thursday morning at ten o'clock.

Madelyn and Beanie wanted to take me, especially since it had been recommended so highly by Floyd Ike. I was hesitant, but figured I would try it, so Glenn drove me to Pennsylvania. Gary and Janet went along to help with my bathroom needs. It was July, very hot, and my feet and hands were swollen from my immobility and the heat. We spent Wednesday night at Glenn's parents' home, and the next morning off we went to Baltimore. Beanie has always loved to drive and wanted to take Glenn and me. Madelyn happened to have a pair of adjustable sandals that went on my very fat feet. I wore a sundress, which was the first and last dress I've worn since becoming totally helpless. I found that caring for someone such as myself in a dress was more trouble than it was worth.

We arrived at the church on time. Everyone was very friendly as we entered. There was a ramp on the side of the church for wheelchairs. There was a side room for those who were unable to go up the stairs to the service. The healer would come there to "lay on his hands" after he had done the same for the others in the sanctuary. Glenn and Beanie insisted they could carry me upstairs in the wheelchair. There were at least 20 steep steps with a U-turn landing in the middle. We made it, but I'm sure if we hadn't been in a church, I would have been screaming the whole way.

The service began with about 35 people present. The first 15 minutes were devoted to meditation, then a hymn was sung, scriptures were read and about a 20-minute sermon followed. Then came the healing. There were two men who did the laying on of hands. I don't even remember their names. At this time, everyone went up in front of the altar railing and waited for a healer to come by, much like it is when one takes communion. The man who came to me had mentioned during the service that a girl with cancer had been healed during a service just a few weeks ago. Well, I was expecting to feel exceptionally warm hands as they were put on my head, since that is what Mrs. Ike said she had experienced when she and her husband attended the service with Olga Worral doing the healing. I really didn't feel a thing, but the man told me to pray and meditate for 15 minutes every night at 9:00 when they had a prayer session. (I continued to do that for a couple of months.) There was neither any collection taken nor donations received during or after the service.

The four of us returned to the car and went to what was then Baltimore's newest tourist attraction, Old Harbor. The paths were brick and made the wheelchair ride very rough. I was both afraid of falling forward when going downhill, and afraid the front wheel would get stuck on a raised brick and throw me forward. Everyone tried to reassure me that would not happen, but then none of them had ever experienced that limp feeling. We stayed a few hours and then headed toward home. By that time, my feet were twice the size they normally were, due to my continuous sitting position and the heat. I had Glenn remove the sandals as soon as he loaded me in the car.

Beanie drove us through the Amish section in Lancaster County, where we saw a huge, nearly perfect rainbow. Glenn patted my shoulder and said, "Maybe that means you're going to get better!"

I thought then, "Boy, I wish I could, but things aren't looking very hopeful."

The next day we headed for Blacksburg, and I continued meditating. Within the next two weeks, the swelling had gone out of my hands, for what reason I didn't know, but nothing else seemed to change. I had heard about a woman who had deteriorated in the same fashion as I and then lived seven years with little change. Then her lungs began to fail, and she succumbed to ALS. I thought that would be my only hope. If I were lucky, perhaps before I got too bad, the scientists would come up with a miracle cure.

After a few months passed, a dear friend, Marjean Anthony, told me of a healer from California whom her sister had gone to for a back problem. The sister had been being treated for a degenerative disc, and the pain was about to get her down when she went to Dennis Adams who was in Cincinnati at the time. She got immediate relief. So, when Marjean's mother was diagnosed with thyroid cancer, Marjean's sister put their parents on a plane to Kansas City, where Dennis Adams happened to be healing at the time. Marjean was very upset with her sister's hasty decision, because she thought her mother should have followed the doctors' advice and had the surgery immediately. Marjean really wasn`t hopeful, but she told me that if her mother improved, then I had better consider going to this man, too. I told her I would if her mother's trip proved successful.

A couple of weeks went by, and her mother went into the hospital for surgery. She asked the surgeon to do a biopsy first before removing the thyroid, but after taking a look at her previous x-rays he insisted that the cancer had already spread to the lymph glands and surgery had to be done as soon as possible. As it turned out, all tests came back negative, with many puzzled physicians. When Marjean told me of her good news, I immediately asked if the cancer had been misdiagnosed, but everyone had assured her that there was simply no way an x-ray could get mixed up with the method that is used in the hospitals today. So, my next step was to call Dennis Adams' office in California. His secretary took my name and number and told me that Dennis would call back. More than a week passed, and I had not heard from him, so I called again. Then I was told that he no longer scheduled individual healing sessions, but was holding seminars on self-healing, with good results. The closest one to us was to be held in Cleveland the first weekend in December.

This wasn't exactly what I was looking for, but the secretary sounded so positive about the whole concept I had her send me the information. The pamphlet arrived, and the cost was $250 per person, with a $50 down payment, $300 without the preregistration fee. Well, again I was game. I immediately sent in $50, along with a letter asking for information on lodging facilities in the area and if there would be any charge for Glenn since he would have to be with me at all times. Weeks went by, and I received no reply. Finally, the time for the seminar was fast approaching, so I called his California office once again. Luckily he answered the phone, and the more I talked with him the more I lost my enthusiasm. He told me that Glenn would also have to pay $250 to be with me, and he didn't know if I should attend since I would need assistance at all times. He thought I might distract everyone else attending the seminar. He would do no individual healing at the seminar, and the weekend retreat was a self-healing, positive-thinking event. He added that I certainly would not get up and walk from such a seminar. Then I inquired as to whether he had ever healed a person with ALS? His reply was "No," because they have never come to me long enough to see if I could help them."

When Glenn came home from work that evening, we discussed the situation, and we both decided that it wasn't my attitude that needed help. So, the next day I was back on the computer writing for my $50 refund. Another good idea down the tube! I did receive my refund, along with the name of a woman who healed in California. I guess my heart wasn't into flying to California to some person I had never heard anything about.

During the time I was trying to find out about Dennis Adams, my sister had had another suggestion. She had been listening to a faith healer on TV. She and Beanie were so amazed over the instant miraculous healing, they wanted me to write to him. So I did, even though I really wasn't convinced that someone would be able to throw away my wheelchair in a matter of minutes, and I would return to normal. Glenn and I then watched his show one Sunday morning. Glenn remarked that it seemed like he was an arthritis specialist!

Weeks passed, and I received no reply to my letter. Perhaps he is a great healer, but I later heard that he would get all the information on a person either before the program started or through letters the person had written to him before attending a healing service. Then, when he called the person's name out, in front of thousands to ask if he had ever met or talked with him or her before, the answer was always, "No." The audience would then be amazed at his 'psychic power.' It was also stated that he would go prepared with a van with wheelchairs he offered to those who showed difficulty walking. Once his wife had quizzed them, he called them to the front for healing. They, in turn, would rise up and walk from their wheelchairs. I then decided that the reason I had never received a letter was the fact that ALS was not something he could handle. Maybe I'm wrong. My letter may have gotten lost because I've never gotten any requests for donations!

Chapter 12

A Star is Born

I have never been much of a daytime TV buff, but to pass the time during the morning hours I often watched the *Today Show* to stay up on the news. The more I watched different news programs, the more irritated I became. Soon after Rock Hudson, the movie star whom I always enjoyed, died from AIDS, every news program would indicate how different organizations were raising large sums of money for AIDS research. Even the government was increasing the allotment for AIDS research. I don't deny that such things should be done, but why had ALS been around for nearly 45 years without nearly so much research having been done? It seemed that little progress had been made in all that time. I called several places to verify my thinking and found my assumption was correct.

For the year 1985, the government designated $108 million for AIDS research and barely $3 million for ALS research. I supposed someone like the President would have to be stricken with ALS before more attention would be given to such a cause. I came to the conclusion that research is based on numbers, and that the 5,000 a year that are victimized with ALS had to depend on a miracle from the few dedicated researchers who are working on the disease. My hope of that happening in my lifetime was barely a glimmer at this point. In order to vent my anger, I told Glenn I was going to write to the *Today Show* and to *Hour Magazine*. After a week and a half passed, I received a phone call from the *Today Show* office in Washington, DC. The young lady who called, Chris Johnson, was very friendly and sympathetic concerning my thoughts. She had called to see if I would be willing to appear on a segment of the show, especially for people who write to the show for one reason or another. I later found out that many letters are received daily, but just a few are picked to go on the air.

After Chris reassured me that there wouldn't be much to taping me, I agreed to do it. When she called, I talked to her on the speaker phone. Gary was with me with a pen and paper to take down all the details. She gave us an idea of what I should say and said that I had 30 seconds to say it. She told me to memorize what I wanted to say, and she and the camera crew would be coming to Blacksburg to film me the following week. After I hung up the phone, both Gary and I felt surprised and elated over such an event. Janet was working as a sales clerk at a small clothing store at the time, so when she came home that evening and we told her of the phone call, she, too, was excited. "A national TV star. Wow!"

Glenn was out of town, so Gary made a yellow star out of construction paper and printed my name on it and taped it to our bedroom door. He told me that was the star's dressing room! When Glenn returned home that Friday night from working in the soybean fields all week, he immediately took his suitcase to our bedroom and noticed the star. "What is this for?" he asked. I then explained, and he just smiled broadly and said, "Oh, no, when is this going to be?"

Two weeks passed, and because of a flood in Roanoke and the arrival of Prince Charles and Princess Diana in the US, there were not enough NBC cameramen to come to small town Blacksburg.

After two weeks of waiting, everyone around me was getting mighty tired of hearing me say my piece! Finally, Chris arranged for a camera crew from the local NBC station in Roanoke to come down to film me, and she flew into Roanoke from Washington. The morning of the filming, Glenn took me to the hairdresser so I would look good for my TV debut. Everyone stayed home from their various jobs that day to watch the unusual event about to happen right in our own home! Three people arrived in the TV station's car about half an hour later than scheduled. There was no time to waste, because Chris had to catch a 3 o'clock flight to return to Washington. My speech was the following:

> I am not a celebrity like Rock Hudson, but I share the same feelings as he had. My physician also gave me the death sentence. I wish someone would do for ALS what he did for AIDS. Within just six months, ALS, or Lou Gehrig's Disease, made me totally dependent on three of my family members. This disease, for which there is no cure, strikes nearly 5,000 citizens a year in this nation. Because of the lack of funds and publicity, not nearly enough research is being done.

After the taping for the national show was finished, the local news show interviewed me while I was in the wheelchair in the backyard. I thought I was absolutely terrible; but when it came out that evening they had cut the bad parts out, and it wasn't nearly so bad as I was anticipating. The tape for the *Today Show* aired nearly two and a half weeks later. It ended the show with a commentator stating that Lou Gehrig, David Niven and New York Senator Jacob Javits had also been stricken with ALS. He added that I was right: there is no cure in sight.

That evening the local TV news ran another short section of the previous taping plus a rerun of the article that had aired on the *Today Show* that morning. I received a postcard from *Hour Magazine*, a CBS morning show, stating they would research the subject. Well, that was the last I heard from them, and, I might say, the last I watched the show.

The letter I had written to the *Today Show* caused me to receive even more publicity. A good friend of mine in Roanoke, Cal Cranor, decided to call the *Roanoke Times* newspaper, the largest paper in the area, and tell them of my fight for more research for ALS. The paper was interested in doing an article and sent a very friendly, personable reporter to interview me. Her name was Debbie Mead, and she came to visit me several times before she wrote a very lengthy and accurate article. It appeared in the paper on a Saturday morning, with pictures taken by a local photographer, Gene Dalton. As a result of that article, two other victims of ALS in the Roanoke area who shared my feelings contacted me. Later, I received calls from someone in Blacksburg whose sister had the disease, and from a young man whose mother lived in Maryland and had had the disease for 16 years. He had sent the article to her, and she had a young friend write me a letter. Years earlier she had received snake venom, a treatment I'm sure wasn't approved by FDA, but possibly it contributed to slowing the nerve cell deterioration. I had never heard of the venom clinic, or I probably would have gotten in line to try it!

I have always enjoyed talking with people, and hearing from these people gave me a satisfying feeling, in a sense, perhaps just knowing that I wasn't alone fighting for a normal life again, which was beginning to look like an impossible dream. One afternoon, I received a telephone call from a young college student who had viewed the *Today Show* the morning that my story appeared, with my name and town flashed across the bottom of the screen. It was Heather, who was majoring in journalism at Virginia Tech, and when she had seen my story on TV she had been surprised that I was from Blacksburg. She asked me if I would be willing to have her interview me for an article to be printed in the college paper. I certainly was glad to oblige. After talking with her, I found that she was not at all comfortable about her self-inflicted assignment! She was doing it for a grade in her journalism class, so before coming to see me she talked to her professor, who told her that he wasn't sure he could handle such an assignment.

Heather was quite apprehensive about how she would talk to me, but after we talked for a while, her nervous-ness left and she found that even though someone can't move, it doesn't change the fact that one is still a human being and has feelings just as someone who can walk. Heather was a very nice person, and she wrote a very well researched article that appeared in the next edition of the *Collegiate Times*.

Later in that school year, I read about a group of young college students on campus who raised money for ALS research. I'm sure if it hadn't been for Heather's article that would not have happened. On the *Today Show* one morning, they were talking to Ann Landers, who had been honored because, through her newspaper column, she was able to encourage the government to allocate $100,000 more for cancer research. What she had done was put a form in the newspaper so anyone who wanted to support more cancer research could sign it and send it to their congressman. Because of the tremendous response, Congress did honor the request.

As I sat there in my chair motionless, my mind started turning and I decided to write to "Dear Ann" to see if she would do the same thing for ALS. She wrote back to me and stated she had been lobbying for money for ALS for two years and would continue to plead, nag, cajole, threaten and do whatever is necessary to get it. I certainly hope she does what she said she would. I have never seen the form in the paper to be signed and sent to congressional representatives for more research money for ALS, though.

After my appearance on TV, our pastor, Ric Elliot, who had always given very good, thought-filled sermons, included my situation in his sermon one Sunday morning. This made the congregation more aware of what I was trying to accomplish. For that reason, the campus pastor, Bill King, had a letter typed and copied so everyone could send it to their congressmen, senators and the director of the National Institutes of Health. The letter read as follows:

> *I am writing to solicit your help in finding a cure for a devastating disease, Amyotrophic Lateral Sclerosis. Until a few months ago, I, like most persons, was only vaguely aware of*

ALS, better known as Lou Gehrig`s disease. But then a vibrant, active woman in our community was diagnosed as suffering from ALS. It has been both painful and frustrating to watch this brave woman's body progressively paralyzed by this disease.

I am aware that many persons suffer from other life threatening diseases, and I would hope that research will continue on such high profile diseases as cancer and heart disease. However, it seems to me that ALS deserves a high priority in research funding, because it is one of the most common neuromuscular disorders (3,000-5,000 new cases each year), because it is so devastating, and because 46 years after the death of Lou Gehrig little progress has been made in isolating the cause or cure of ALS.

I request that you use your influence to insure adequate governmental funding for research. Private groups such as the Muscular Dystrophy Association are hard at work doing research, but strong governmental funding is necessary if significant progress is to be made·

Thank you for your support·

Sincerely,

The congregation got a reply back from the National Institute of Neurological and Communicative Disorders and Stroke to assure them that some of our nation's best scientific minds are seeking answers to ALS, and that Federal support of ALS research will continue until this disease is conquered. It all sounds great, but I can tell you, from experience, it is of little immediate comfort to the person suffering from the disease!

My next step was to write to the CBS television show, *60 Minutes*. I was hoping perhaps they could run a segment and interview several victims and their families to show just how severely the disease can change people's lives. I was hoping that it would create public awareness of the disease and of how little is known about it, but that idea was shot down in a hurry. They sent me a letter saying they were sorry they would be unable to air my request, because they receive so many letters and it would be impossible to use all of them.

By the end of 1985, I think, my writing for more support for research had come to an end. I just felt like I had done about all I could do. I had bugged the places that needed to be aware of ALS patients' and their families' problems, so those people and organizations would do what they could, but it didn't seem as if I was able to do any more than just scratch the surface.

Nelda Buss

Chapter 13

The Healers 11

Marjean came often to see me. She was disappointed that my trip to see Dennis Adams had never worked out. One day in November, when she came to visit she brought a copy of an article from that month's issue of *American Health*. Her neighbor, whom I did not know at the time, and to whom I'll be forever grateful, had given an article that discussed psychic healing to Marjean to give to me. After Marjean left, I read the article, several times. It mentioned two healers who were scientifically tested and found to have special power that radiated from their hands and for that reason had been able to heal many people. The two who were mentioned were Olga Worrall and Dean Kraft. I knew Olga had died, and all the article gave for Dean Kraft's address was New York.

As Janet, Gary and I sat around the kitchen table discussing the article, I told them I was going to try to call Dean Kraft. They were both in agreement, because they both knew nothing else was going to improve my con-dition. I called my friend with whom I had worked before I was forced to go on disability. She was a conference programming assistant and often made out-of-state phone calls. I knew she had a lot of phone books, among them the New York City directory. I had no idea whether this Dean Kraft was in the city or possibly somewhere in the state of New York. When my friend checked the city phone book, she said there was just one Dean Kraft in the book and warned me that the directory she had was two years old. Janet and Gary were still at the table listening to my conversation. After hanging up, I said, "God must be looking out for me."

Again, I picked up my mouth-stick from the cup and called the number she had given me. He had an answering service. I asked the person on the other end if this were the Dean Kraft who did psychic healing. Her reply was, "I guess, he does something like that!"

I wasn't too optimistic after that reaction, but I left my number so he could return my call. Four days had passed before his wife, Rochelle, called me from Los Angeles, California, where (as I later found out) he also did healing. As I talked with Rochelle, explaining my situation and telling her that the doctors gave me no hope, she assured me that Dean would be glad to see me, since those people left with no hope at all made up most of his business. She said he would see me the very next weekend, but because the *Today Show* filming was scheduled that week and it seemed just too quick, I needed more time to think about it. I set up an appoint-ment in three weeks.

The closest place I could see Dean would be in his New York office, where he "treated" people Saturdays and Sundays every other weekend. She gave me the address. Since Janet and Gary were familiar with New York, Gary was confident that he would have no problem finding it and assured me it was in a very nice area of the city. Before Rochelle hung up the phone, she said she would send me

Dean's autobiography if I would be interested in reading it.
I told her I would.

A few days passed, and I received a small paperback in the
mail entitled *A Portrait of a Psychic Healer.* I was never much
of a reader, I suspect because I was always busy doing work
on the farm and enjoyed being outside better than reading
books. Anyway, I read Dean's book in two evenings. It all
sounded so good—in fact, too good to be true! I hoped
that maybe with some luck something miraculous would
happen to me as had happened to so many fortunate
people in his book.

Three weeks passed, and we were ready to take another
long trip, the first since July. On December 6, 1985, I was
dressed, fed and put into the car. Along with Glenn, Gary
and Janet, I sped off toward Pennsylvania. Before leaving,
I had decided I would not eat or drink much so that
perhaps we would not have to make a rest stop for me to
use the bedpan. Glenn drove and Gary sat behind me in
the car so he could move my bottom every hour or two.
The pain or uncomfortable feeling became almost
unbearable. When you lose the use of your extremity
muscles with ALS, you lose the bounce resistance that you
never knew you had when you were well, but you never
lose the feeling as one does when they are paralyzed from
a spinal injury. I would suspect that is why I never ended
up with bedsores, because I could feel when it felt like the
bone started to come through the skin. Anyway, my
bladder held up the whole trip, and I spared everyone from
getting out in the cold weather to set up the latrine!

We arrived at Glenn's folks' home with no problem and
spent the night. The next day, we all ate an early lunch and
left the Buss' at 11:13 a.m. for my two o'clock appointment
in the city. I had mixed emotions about the whole thing.
1 thought, "What kind of wild goose chase am I taking

everyone on now?" I had no idea what this man was going to look like. Was he going to have a robe on? What was he going to do with me? I don't remember the conversation that took place between Gary (now the driver), Glenn and Janet in the back seat, but I was probably in such deep thought that I did very little talking. We arrived around 1:30, having had no problem finding the small office on 37th Street.

We rang the bell and waited for Rochelle to open the door, which she did after checking through a speaker to see who was outside. This was a new experience for me. In Blacksburg, oftentimes, the doors are unlocked and you just yell, "Come in." I have found city living to be a much more defensive living! Glenn and Gary maneuvered me, in the wheelchair, up the narrow three-step entryway. We all met Rochelle immediately. She was a very striking, good-looking, vibrant person in her early thirties. Gary and Janet took the car to a parking garage, which turned out to be about a $9 expense! While they were doing that, Glenn completed a form that Rochelle had given him to fill out for me.

Questions on the form included why you were there, where you had been diagnosed and when you had last seen your doctor. To the last question I had to answer January 18, 1985, because I had not gone back to the doctor after I left the University of Virginia hospital. I wasn't about to pay someone $35 to tell me I was a little worse than I was before when I could tell that myself. The form concluded with a statement for me to sign saying that I had exhausted all medical avenues and that the treatment I was about to receive would not be guaranteed to be effective. Glenn read everything to me and then signed it for me.

Soon, Dean came out from his small office, introduced himself to Glenn and me, and told us to come on in. He was a very friendly, short, dark-haired young man, dressed in a dark pair of pants and a plain knit shirt; certainly nothing out of the ordinary! The door to his office was so narrow that the wheelchair would not fit through, so Glenn picked me up under my arms and carried me about four feet to the blue leather portable table that sat along the painted wall. He laid me down and placed a pillow from the sofa that sat against the other wall under my knees. I could not bear to straighten my knees because of the joint pain. Dean then asked Glenn to sit down. Closing the door, he proceeded to ask whether I was on any medication and whether I had tried to get into any experimental programs working with trial drugs for ALS. After I recounted my many attempts to combat the disease, he suggested that Glenn wait out in the waiting room while he worked on me.

He then began doing his thing. He sat at the end of the table where my head was lying on a pillow. His hands seemed very warm as he held them about a half-inch above the skin above my right eye and the right side of my head. When he then moved his hands to my shoulders, I felt a vibration that made me think his whole body must be shaking. Next, though, he walked around to my left side and placed his hands on my arms and legs, and I noticed that only his hands vibrated, and that was barely visible.

What was so remarkable was that he carried on a conversation with me the whole 15 to 20 minutes that I was there. I told him about the *Today Show* that I had appeared on just days before seeing him. He told me of a documentary he planned to do for TV. I told him that if he helped me, perhaps I could be part of that. He said that I certainly would be, and he was very optimistic that he would be able to help me. He told me that doctors only know what is in the medical books and that he had helped most of his patients—more than 70 percent.

Glenn then came in the room to get me. He took the pillow from beneath my knees, lifted my head up, sat me up and carried me back to the wheelchair. Dean told me that first he would work at getting the disease into remission and then start working on regaining the muscle loss. He said he would have to work with me six weeks before he would know for sure whether he could help or not. He told Glenn that he would like to see me the next day if at all possible, because the more "hands on," the better it would be for me. So, Glenn paid Rochelle, who takes care of all of the bookwork, and set up another appointment for 5:15 the next day.

Chapter 14

First Signs of Hope

As Dean worked on me, I could feel my lungs rattling; and as I was waiting for Glenn to pay the bill, I had to cough phlegm up several times, something I had not been able to do for months. Gary and Glenn loaded me into the car and were glad to hear that I was going to make another trip to the city the next day. They were hopeful. We then drove to Pennsylvania on Rt. 80 and stopped in for a good sausage dinner with Madelyn and Beanie, who were eagerly awaiting my arrival to hear of my experience. As I was wheeled into their kitchen, my nose began to run due to the cold night air. Glenn got a Kleenex and I blew my nose, but with more power than I had been able to muster for several months. I looked at Glenn and he at me. We both grinned as we realized a change had occurred already. In fact, Glenn told me to try it again, just to check it out! It was such a slight change, the more we talked about it, the more we were wondering if it were just our imagination. We drove back to the Buss' home and spent the night.

The next day, we ate our breakfast and got ready to return to NYC. We visited with Glenn's brother, Robin, over lunch. Since Rosanne, his wife, was still in the hospital after giving birth to their son, Steven, he had lunch with all of us. Then Glenn's Aunt Edith and Uncle Elvin came to visit a little before we took off for NYC once again. We left at 2:45 to make our 5:15 appointment. We arrived on time, but because so many people were waiting to see Dean, I did not go in with him until 6:40. He worked on me about a half hour in much the same manner as he had the day before, except he had me meditate for about 15 minutes, thinking of a clear, calm lake. Again I could feel the phlegm in my lungs loosen. As Glenn sat me up, I again was able to cough.

Each "zap," as Dean calls them, lasts about 12 to 13 minutes, which costs $100. The first day I had one zap; the next day two. During our chatting, Dean again told me that he wanted me for his documentary and said the filming would take place within four to six weeks. He assured me he would let me know just what to expect and what type of taping would be done, specifically whether it would be an interview or a story-type filming. He also told me that in Los Angeles he was treating someone who works for CBS's *60 Minutes*, and he would give me the man's name and address so that my letter would get to the right person. I gave him my picture, which he had asked for the day before, and the newspaper article from the *Roanoke Times*. He was very pleased to get them, because that would give him something to relate to when he sees me. I'm not sure if he does psychic healing from a distance or not. He told me to be sure to come back in two weeks, at which time he would give me two sessions back to back. I left feeling encouraged and expecting to go every other week for a long time, but hopeful that some progress might be seen in six weeks. Glenn and I decided that we would come back in two weeks, and schedule two treatments on Saturday and two on Sunday.

Having left our $200 check with Rochelle, we headed again for Bath, PA, to spend the night with Glenn's parents. We left for Virginia the next morning, all feeling more hope than we had come with, but still not sure it was possible to get any worthwhile improvement in my condition.

I remember when I first came home from the hospital and was swamped with company. I told Glenn then that I hoped they wouldn't forget about me when things began to get much worse. Human nature being what it is, some indeed had stopped visiting, certainly not because they forgot about me, but everyone settles into their daily routine and life goes on. Now that I look back on some of last year's visitors, I have to chuckle. Some never wanted to speak to me when I was well, but came running when they heard I was going to die. Then when I started to recover, I never heard from them again. Then there were those who came only to find out what I was doing in New York! Of course, there were many who stuck by me no matter what—those I have to consider my true-blue friends.

One couple who always came to visit were Nick and Arlene Hudgins. After Dorothy's husband became a victim of a stroke that incapacitated him, Dorothy was unable to set up visitors for me. I assured everyone that I was doing fine, and I hated to bother anyone with such a chore. Arlene nonetheless insisted that she would schedule the visitors so that I would not get too bored. I know that when you are recovering from anything, you must keep your spirits high and my company helped me do that.

In retrospect, however, there is one thing I would do differently. If I had to go through the first three months of my trips to Dean again, I don't think I would tell anyone except a few very close friends. My experience was that when I did tell some of the people, almost all said they would not try it themselves and certainly wouldn't encourage me too much because of the potential disappointment of seeing no results for my efforts. I soon was able to tell each person's reaction by reading facial expressions. In fact, it soon became a source of entertainment for me. Some who knew what I was doing would ignore the whole issue, because they were afraid to talk about it!

Despite a lot of outside negativity, my family still wanted me to continue my trips to New York. So, on December 19 and 20, I spent an hour with Dean each day. Other than the fact that my lungs seemed to have more activity when he worked on me, I saw no other change. He gave me a total of four "treatments," which cost a total of $400. Then he told us that in order for me to tell if he could help me, I would have to have a total of 30 treatments. With such serious illnesses as mine, sometimes as high as 50 treatments are necessary before any results are evident. Dean further suggested that I take the extensive treatments in Florida, where he does some healing in his home. Instead, because of the problems with the care I would need on a long trip and the expense for everyone's food and lodging, we decided to stick to New York.

Before we left, Dean told me to meditate two times a day, once in the morning and once in the evening. My meditation was to consist of picturing a calm lake with no ripples, because each ripple represents a thought and you want to clear your mind of all thoughts. After doing that for five minutes, I was to imagine a bright white light going around my body and try to feel the heat from the light penetrating into the parts of my body that needed healing. That part took me about 15 minutes, because my whole body needed repairing, and it took a lot of concentration to get around my body several times. Then the last thing I was supposed to do was to imagine myself doing something that I would like to do, such as walking, sewing, cooking, etc.

As always, Dean was very encouraging. He told me of some of his more recent healings, from cancer to bringing someone out of a coma. As Glenn was about to pick me up from the table, Dean told him that he felt that 1986 would be a better year than 1985. We spent Christmas with hope, but also a lot of uncertainty. My Christmas gifts were things for the home. After all, what do you buy someone when she is unable to do anything and is doomed to die!

When January 3 rolled around, Gary and Janet drove me to Pennsylvania. Glenn was unable to go, because he had to teach during the winter quarter and time did not permit him to leave. With Gary doing the driving, we made the trip in just a little more than 6.5 hours. We stopped at a fast food place, where they went in for the food. We ate as we drove. Janet fed me. My fast food order was always chicken pieces, since they were easier for her to feed me. I was quite careful to chew well, because I had a fear of choking and not being able to cough very well. She was always considerate, giving me small bites and keeping a glass of water with a straw handy just in case I needed it.

My bottom needed to be moved several times as we rode, but other than that I found the trips to be enjoyable— certainly more than sitting at home! We stayed again with Glenn's parents, where we were fed generously. The next day Gary and Janet drove me to Madelyn and Beanie's house for lunch, and we left around 3:00 to go to New York for my 5:30 appointment with Dean.
Dean worked with me for two hours. We went back to Pennsylvania and then did the same thing the next day. During my time with Dean, I probably spent an hour chatting each day and an hour meditating. The two-hour trip to New York was about all my bottom could take. It

was so painful that I couldn't wait to be put in the wheelchair when I got to Dean's office. Then when I lay on the table for two hours, my tailbone would hurt.

After I got back to the Buss' home and Gary had propped me in a comfortable position, I found that sleeping did not come easily. Gary was also nursing a sore throat, so between that and getting up and turning me during the night to make me more comfortable, he certainly did not have a fun-filled night. Although weary, we made the trip back to Virginia just fine. That night Glenn gave me a shower and gave me my daily exercises. He said it seemed to him that my joints were moving more freely.

The next Thursday, when Janet gave me my arm exercises in the chair, I think we were both in a state of disbelief when I didn't yell as she put my arms through their range of motion. I remember looking at Janet and telling her, "It's a miracle!" My joints still hurt a little, but not nearly so much as before. In fact, she was able to do each arm ten times, whereas before that she would stop after four times because she knew it was painful and she hated to put me through the agony.

When Gary was called to the scene, he immediately wanted to lift up my foot to straighten my leg and check the pain in my knees. To our amazement, they didn't hurt! Before, I would have screamed.

Chapter 15

Dean ~ January and February 1986

January 17 rolled around, and we were on the road again. We made our usual stop in Pennsylvania, and on Saturday Madelyn and Beanie were again ready to take Janet, Gary and me to the city. As soon as Gary had put me on the table and made me comfortable, Dean closed the door behind him and began asking me if I had seen any changes. My largest noticeable change was, of course, less pain. He then took the pillow out from under my knees and asked me to raise my feet off the table with my knees bent. To my surprise, I could lift them about five inches. The next test was moving each finger, and I was able to move one finger a tiny bit.

Dean was overwhelmed with excitement, so much so he had to call Gary back into the office to have me perform— then Rochelle, then Gary and Janet. After all the joy and excitement subsided, everybody left the office and Dean continued to work on me for the next two hours. After we left his office, they wheeled me down the street into a

2e222ф222222222222

Chinese restaurant where we celebrated my birthday, which seemed to be a little bit better than the year before! But I must say there were a lot of questions running through my mind. Could I have moved my feet like that before if I had tried? And maybe even one finger—was it better than before? To me, the improve-ment was ever so slight. How could I ever get back to normal at this rate?

I know everyone else had those same questions in mind, but nobody mentioned it because they all realized the value of a positive attitude. We drove the two-hour trip back to Pennsylvania and went to bed about 11:00. My tailbone hurt so badly from lying on the table for that length of time that getting comfortable seemed almost impossible. As a result, I had to disturb Gary's sleep very often.

Glenn's parents live in a big farmhouse with the bed-rooms upstairs, but in order to accommodate me they had been kind enough to turn two downstairs rooms into bedrooms. That way I could sleep in one room and someone else could sleep in the next room so they could hear me if I needed help. Gary was the one designated to be on call for that night, and since we had to get up at 4:30 the next morning, little rest was acquired!

A little after 5:00 a.m., Gary was driving Glenn's father, Janet and me into the city on a very rainy morning. Because my tailbone hurt so badly when I was on the table, we had decided to take foam along to help soften the spot where it came in contact with the table. Since it was very early and I had gotten barely three hours of sleep, Dean was very quiet through most of the treatment, but even as tired as I felt I was not able to sleep. We had left the city by 9:30, and most of the Buss family was there to help celebrate my birthday. We enjoyed a pretty birthday cake that was prepared by Mrs. Buss. After everyone else left, we all were a bit tired, and by ten o'clock I was put to bed and the lights went out. I slept till 2:30 a.m., when my hip woke me up, and I had to call Janet, my helper nominated for the night, to try to alleviate the pain somehow. She decided to try a thicker piece of foam under my hip, and to my surprise I went right back to sleep and slept till 6:00 a.m., the best sleep I had had in a week!

After leaving for Virginia that morning, we ran into some snow. Luckily, it snowed hard for only about a half-hour, and we had clear sailing the rest of the way home. After eating dinner, Glenn gave me my bath and put me through my exercise routine. He noticed that my legs were definitely better. He then put me in the wheelchair and took me out to a swivel rocker in the living room to watch TV. To my amazement, I found I could turn myself with my feet—not much or fast, but it was some-thing I could not have done before. That surely made me feel even more hopeful!

Two weeks went by, and it was time once again to hit the road for New York. This trip Paula and Russ decided to fly into the Newark Airport on Saturday. The weather was good, but the forecast was calling for snow. Luckily, the weatherman's prediction never did materialize. On Saturday morning, Janet and Gary got me washed, dressed and fed, loaded me into the car, and we were on the road again by 8:00 a.m. At the airport, Paula and Russ just came out to the loading zone as we pulled up, so as soon as we got everything and everybody into the car we headed for the Holland Tunnel so they could see the Statue of Liberty. This was their first trip into the city, so Gary wanted to show them a few things.

The first thing to see was the traffic! Being used to driving in the city from when he lived there before, Gary was not a bit shy about the gas and brake pedals, which he seemed to be using simultaneously! Our first stop was in Brooklyn to show them where Gary used to live, which was not too impressive. I guess you can't expect much when it only costs $700 a month rent. We drove through Chinatown and back to Manhattan. I really hated that they had to drag me around with them all over. I felt they could have seen a lot more if they hadn't had to take the time to fool with me, but they didn't seem to mind.

Our next stop was to find a parking lot near the World Trade Center. Gary got me out and put me into the wheelchair, after which we walked about three blocks and were able to buy a ticket for $2.75 each to go to the 107th floor to view the city. It was a very nice panoramic view; I think we all enjoyed it. Next was a visit to Macy's, somewhere I had never been before. Often while I was at Dean's for the two hours, the others would spend the time shopping, and I, of course, never had the opportunity. My thoughts about shopping certainly were not what they had once been, anyway. I remember many a time as I sat in the car in front of shopping centers while Glenn would run in to pick something up, I would wonder what the sense was to be buying so much. Monetary things seemed unimportant in my situation.

Well, anyway, Paula and Russ took me into Macy's, while Janet and Gary parked the car. It seemed as though we spent more time on the elevator going from floor to floor than anything else, but it was fun. From there we went on to Mamma Leone's where Paula and Russ treated me to my belated birthday dinner. It was good, but hardly worth the $108 we paid for five pasta dinners! Our next stop was Dean's office, which was 15 blocks away. Gary always tried to make my life exciting, and speeding with the wheelchair was one way of accomplishing it. I didn't have a strap to hold me in, because if the operator of the wheelchair were gentle it was not necessary. Needless to say, I felt very insecure when I could not hold on with my hands. On the way down to 37th Street, I yelled at Gary a few times to slow down, but he seemed to think he had everything in control, as usual! As I was being pushed hastily through an intersection and bumped up onto the sidewalk, I had a look of fear on my face that must have prompted a lady who stopped Janet and informed her that she should tell me to hold onto the arms of the wheelchair. She said it in a tone of voice that led Janet to think that she thought I didn't have enough sense to do it myself! Janet's reply was quick: "She would if she could!" That gave us all a big laugh.

When I arrived at Dean's office, I told him of the episode and he just said, "We'll get you so you'll be able to hold on." After he had worked on me for two hours, Gary loaded me up and we all arrived back at the Buss' home safely. Even though it was a rush trip for Paula and Russ, we all enjoyed it. We took them back to the airport for an 11:30 flight and sat in a parking area along the Hudson River eating a packed lunch and trying to kill time, since my appointment with Dean wasn't until 3:45 that afternoon.

Being the naive country girl that I am, I had my eyes opened to another kind of life. We sat and watched the gay prostitutes while we ate our lunch. My first thought was one of fear; I wanted Gary to quickly lock the car doors. I certainly did not feel comfortable eating my lunch there, but after a while I did not feel threatened. As Gary told me, "They aren't after you!"

Well, it became very entertaining. We watched as four or five prissy-looking young men walked up and down the long parking area. One fellow had on a jock strap under his white see-through tights. It certainly didn't leave much to the imagination. Another one had a matching bright green hat and scarf, which were adjusted frequently with very feminine gestures. We sat there at least an hour, but no one had any takers during that time. As we were about to leave, the one in the white tights decided to relieve himself by standing on the pier and polluting the Hudson River even more than it already was.

We then left that area and went into a better area of the city, passing through many sections that were not too prosperous. I feel very sorry for the many people we saw along the way. What a way to live! But to them it probably is just their way of life, and if they had to live the way we live, they would not like it either. We then went to Dean's at 3:00, only to find that he was not well and would not be able to treat me. Gary and Janet took me into the office anyway, so I could use the bathroom.

Back to Pennsylvania we drove, then got up the next morning for the trip to Virginia. During the following week, I was able to press the shift key on the computer with one finger and my left wrist was able to lift my left hand up from the bed about two inches. Then when I returned home from New York after my next trip, I noticed immediately that I could lift my feet up about three more inches when I sat on the rocking chair. It never ceased to amaze me what strength I would gain after seeing Dean. Gary and Janet continued doing exer-cises with me an hour a day. I certainly didn't enjoy them, but I knew I would have to work hard at it if I were ever to regain my strength.

Pain was always present in the joints during the exercises. It felt as if they were placing my extremities in a position that was impossible for any arm or leg! Our neighbor, Mary Jenkins, came over and presented me with a sponge ball taken from a bottle washer, just as soon as she heard I was to squeeze a sponge ball to help my finger muscles develop. The therapeutic putty and the "nerf ball" were entirely too hard for my fingers at that stage. In fact those fingers barely moved the very pliable sponge that Mary gave me. I tried hard, but not much seemed to happen. With Gary's constant "cracking the whip," I did more than I probably would have done on my own.

During the summer of 1985 our friends from eastern Virginia, Ellie and Joe Miklos, heard about my illness. It was a matter of disbelief to them, since they had spent some time with us the previous summer, and I had been perfectly healthy. They heard the news as they were about to hike a portion of the Appalachian Trail. They both had a very fulfilling time on the trail, but Ellie said she thought of me often. When that summer ended, Ellie returned to her job teaching third grade at a local elementary school. She immediately told her class about me and suggested that they adopt me as a pen pal. I soon began to receive letters from all of her pupils. It was fun reading them. Of course, someone had to help me turn the papers.

On February 8, 1986, Ellie drove the five-hour trip to our house to visit and to videotape me so the children could see me. With her she brought along a tape of the children that she had recorded during the previous week. Each one of them had a chance to say something about themselves. It was a real treat for me. I watched it several times and still look at it occasionally. Some of the children were very humorous.

Well, that was the beginning of home movies for me! Ellie taped the beginnings of my progress. Even though there wasn't much action, it was better than ever predicted. I was able to sit forward a little when I sat in a chair, I could move a few fingers and I was able to slide my stocking feet up and down on a satin sheet when lying on the bed. My feet were very swollen, and my toes did not move yet. Ellie said they flunked the test. She returned to her job the next

Monday morning, and I continued to hear from the children until their summer vacation began.

On February 24, I could clasp my hands together, twist my wrists and bring my hands up to my chest. What an accomplishment! I found out I could do that while Glenn was away on a business trip. When he returned, the first thing I did was show him my new trick, and he was quite excited. By February 28, I was ready to go to New York once again. My back had been bothering me for about six weeks. I had gotten two different pills from my family doctor, but neither seemed to help. It seemed to hurt only after I would sleep for four hours, at which time the pain was so intense I just couldn't sleep. I finally told Dean about it. He said he had worked on a lot of bad backs, and he would work on mine. He helped me turn on my side and did just that. Within a week, my back pain was a thing of the past!

While I was in with Dean for my two-hour session, Madelyn, Beanie, Gary and Janet decided to go uptown to shop for a camera for Beanie. They were so proud of themselves, because they found a street with meter parking and only a few cars were parked there. They put their money in and shopped the next hour and a half. But when they came back to the car they found a ticket on the windshield! They looked up, and sure enough there were signs that said no parking between 4:00 p.m. and 7:00 p.m. Gary and Janet felt bad, because they had told Beanie it was okay to park there, so Gary was planning to pay the parking ticket. On the way home, we stopped at a hamburger place, where we were eating in the car, because I still didn't like going inside to eat. For some reason, Gary decided to check Beanie's license plate number against the number written on the ticket. Well, to everyone's delight, the meter maid had made a mistake, and there was one number wrong! So, no one paid the ticket, and Beanie probably didn't drive that car into the city again for another six months. He considered it his 'hot' car!

The next day Gary, Janet and I headed south again. The next week, I found I could lift my feet a few inches higher, and I ate my first sandwich by myself. I held it with two hands; it was messy, but I did it!

Chapter 16

Dean - March and April 1986

In March, we made another video of my progress. It wasn't a lot, but a definite improvement over the last taping was obvious. Each time we did a taping, we would make a copy and give it to Dean. I continued to go to him every two weeks for a two-hour session each time. Each time, I would see some improvement. Sometimes I felt a bit depressed, because I thought I should be getting better faster. Then I would have to remember what it had been like just a month or two before and begin to think more positively.

On Good Friday, everyone was back on the road to Pennsylvania again. We arrived at the Buss' a little after 4:00. Gary and Janet ate a quick sandwich, got back in our car and drove up to RIT to visit their friends. Glenn and I were ready by 10:00 the next morning to go up to Madelyn and Beanie's. We had a small lunch, and then by 11:45 we were back in the car for our New York trip. We reached

Dean's in time for my 2:00 appointment. Glenn put me on the table and went into Rochelle's office where she taped an interview with him with their new mini-video camera. Because of the lack of good lighting, I was not filmed. Dean worked with me for two hours once again. He was excited about his movie script being completed and told me that he wanted me to play myself in the movie. What a thing to look forward to!

Dean was pleased with the progress I had been making. He was impressed with the video we had made at home. It showed what I could do at home, which was much more than what was visible at his office. I showed him how I could put the footrest on my wheelchair up with my right foot. I could see myself improving a little each day. Improvement seemed slow, but all good things take time. I meditated about an hour of the two-hour session. I asked him if he would see Ed Mitchell, an ALS victim from Roanoke. Dean said he would be glad to see him, and that Ed could call him in Florida to set something up.

Dean worked a lot on my head once again, along with my right arm. My right arm was a lot weaker than my left, even with the extra exercise I tried to give it. With a lot of exercising ahead of me, Dean was sure that I would be back 100 percent. As soon as my arms became strengthened enough to support my body, I would need to get braces and begin walking with a walker. I was exercising at least two hours every day, but it takes a lot of time for the muscles to get stronger.

After I got finished with Dean, we all went to Joe's Pier 52 for our 25th anniversary dinner. We all enjoyed a good seafood dinner and then returned to Pennsylvania by 10:00 that night. At this point, I could push the wheelchair forward on a smooth surface. I could pick up the sponge ball or stick if I dropped it while I was in the swivel rocker at home. My thumb and first finger were beginning to come closer together. I was using my mouth stick when I watched TV to operate the remote control. Soon, I found I could bend down when I was sitting in the rocker and pick up my mouth stick when I dropped it. This was not done with ease and not always with success, but it was another step. Everything took a lot of concentration and effort, but I knew with time and practice things should get easier.

Meditation and exercise still took up a major part of my morning. To get my muscle strength back, I was going to have to work hard. Nothing was easy, but Gary and Janet helped take the drudgery out of the daily routine. They were always there to help me when I needed it and joked around a lot, so things didn't get boring.

On April 11, Glenn and I left for New York once again. We arrived at his parents' home at 4:00. It was cold all weekend, but we had no rain or snow during our travels. The next day we had a big breakfast before leaving for Madelyn and Beanie's. She had a big lunch for us, including a birthday cake for Glenn. We left for New York about 1:00 to make my 3:15 appointment. When we got in Dean's office, there was a twelve-year-old boy waiting with his father to see Dean. They were very interested in my problem and how I was responding. Dean later told me that the little boy had had brain surgery and chemotherapy treatment, which weakened his muscles on his right side. It was only his second visit, and he was already seeing some improvement.

When I did get in to see Dean, it was nearly 4:00. He took a videotape of me before he began my treatment. He did have me meditate a lot on the lake, the light and on bowling. He showed me the script for his movie, which he hoped to begin filming in September. He said he would have a copy for me the next time I saw him, and I would be playing the part of Pauline. It really did not seem even close to being real at that point! He was pleased with my progress and told me that he thought he could safely say that I no longer had ALS and that I was just fighting the effects from the disease. He then gave me a cassette tape of his energy video, which he had made to sell. He told me to watch it at least once a day. He gave Glenn a little "zap" on his right shoulder in the hope that it would help his long-time injury.

Glenn put me in the wheelchair when I got finished with my healing session, while Beanie went after the car, which was in a parking garage. Madelyn and Glenn decided to take me outside to wait for Beanie. Well, Madelyn was not experienced with helping with the wheelchair, and she didn't manage to hold the front end up as we went down the stairs. I still wasn't strong enough to hold myself in it, and I was sure I would get dumped out on my face. They finally got me on the sidewalk, but not without a blood-curdling yell from my mouth! Everyone came running, but things soon got under control. Whew, was I glad when I was sitting upright once again.

When I look back on that now, it seems pretty funny, but it didn't seem funny to me when it was happening. Trust in the people around you is something that a disabled person must develop, but it is not always easy to do. While we were driving through New York, I would usually see the big pretzels being sold on many of the street corners. I had often thought I would like to have one, so on this trip Glenn bought me one. We kept it until we got back to Madelyn and Beanie's place, and there we all had a taste of the New York pretzel. Yuk—it was awful! It tasted like smoke, I won't ask for another one of those.

Before we left, Beanie brought out a pedal machine he had designed and made for me to use in my exercising. He had put two pedals on a block of wood and even put carpeting on them to make them soft for my feet. They worked like bike pedals. I could turn them after someone put my feet on them, but after one turn my feet would fall off. So Glenn got some rope and tied my feet on the pedals. The first few days that I worked with them, someone had to help turn them, but soon I was able to turn the machine myself. Then I began using it for my arms, too, but again somebody had to tie my hands on the pedals before I could turn them.

My progress seemed slower at this point. I did get a little stronger each time, but it was not as noticeable because it was just building strength onto the muscles I already had. My legs had improved to the point I could do my leg exercises on the bed without the satin. I could kick them out and back much better when I was lying on my side. My arms also were a bit stronger. I noticed that when I brought my hands up together it didn't take as much effort as it first had. It was now Friday, April 18, and I was able to operate the pedals fairly easily, compared to when I had started on Monday. I was hoping that with this new exerciser I would be able to improve a little faster.

On April 26, 1986, Debbie, the reporter from the *Roanoke Times*, and the photographer, Gene Dalton, rode to Pennsylvania with Glenn and me. Debbie was interested in my progress and wanted to write an updated story on me, since I seemed to be getting stronger, and I wasn't supposed to be. On that trip, I was able to cross my feet at the ankles. It always made me feel good when I could do something new. When we got to Allentown, we dropped Debbie and Gene off at the bus station so they could go on into New York and see the sights. Glenn and I went on to his parents' place as we usually did. When we arrived there, we were surprised to see a horse peering out of the barn. It seems their neighbor's son had married a girl with a horse and had no place to keep it. S-o-o-o, they had asked Pop to keep it for them. He said he would. This horse was supposedly a very much-loved animal, but it had been there two weeks and no one had come back to see it. The next morning, Glenn had to hustle to get himself and me ready. It was the weekend that we turned the clocks ahead, so we had one less hour to work with. We got on the road by 11:45 and got into the city right on time for my 2:00 appointment.

Luck was with us! There was a parking place right in front of Dean's office, where Debbie and Gene were waiting for us. When we got into the office, I introduced them to Dean and Rochelle. Dean took Debbie into his office and gave her a brief treatment. She interviewed him for about 15 minutes. Interviews are something that Dean very rarely permits, but after talking with Debbie he felt very good about the coverage she would give the story—and I did, too. After they finished talking, Glenn carried me over to the table, and Gene took several pictures with Dean giving a demonstration of his healing technique. Then they all left to walk the streets while Dean worked on me. When I was finished, Glenn and Debbie had to help me go to the bathroom. Glenn held me while Debbie yanked the pants! When I got put back together, we went to a nice restaurant on 55th Street, where the tab was picked up by the *Roanoke Times*. We all had filet mignon, and Debbie and Gene ordered escargot, so Glenn and I sampled our first snail. It was not bad tasting, but it is not something I'd order for myself. We did thoroughly enjoy our meal, though. We finished eating by 7:00 and headed back to Allentown. We dropped Debbie and Gene off at the Red Roof Inn at the airport exit. The next morning we picked them up at 9:20 and headed for Blacksburg.

Our trip back to Virginia was very enjoyable. We talked about a lot of different things, stopping at McDonald's for lunch and arriving in Blacksburg at 5:00. Getting a bath now wasn't quite as frightening as it had once been, but I was still mighty glad to get back into the wheelchair, where I felt more secure. That night while Glenn was giving me my bath, I noticed my feet went up three inches or so higher than they had the week before. I also found that sometimes I could put the footrests on the wheelchair down with my feet. I could put my right foot over my left at the ankles, but the other way around took a lot of effort.

Chapter 17

Dean - May and June 1986

On May 10, Janet and Gary put me in the car for another trip north. Since it was Mother's Day weekend, Glenn's brothers and their families were all at his parents' home when we arrived. We had a nice visit and all enjoyed the evening meal together. Paula and Russ also called to talk with me to wish me a Happy Mother's Day. By nine o'clock, everyone had left for home and by eleven we were all in bed. Gary decided to just prop two pillows on the left side of my legs and not to put the pillows under my knees as I had been used to doing. I turned on my right side several times during the night and did not have to call Gary out of bed at all to get me comfortable. What an accomplishment! The pillows held the blankets up so I did not get tangled in them when I turned. I always woke up to turn, because it was something that I had to think about when I did it. It was not really easy to do, but if felt so good when I could do it!

The next morning, Gary and Janet got me dressed, and we left to go to New York with Madelyn and Beanie. I took along a letter for Dean, which I had written with two hands. It was legible, and surprisingly it looked very much like my old handwriting. It was a short letter with about five sentences, which took me about 25 minutes to write, but everyone in Dean's office was proud of it. I must say, no one was more proud than I.

When the end of May rolled around, Gary and Janet were ready for a vacation. They planned a trip to Colorado to visit a high-school friend of Gary's. They decided to fly out of Newark Airport, since that was a lot cheaper than flying from Roanoke. So, on the way to my appointment in the city, we dropped them off at the airport, and they began a well-deserved two-week vacation. My progress was slow, but steady. When I was lying on the bed, I was now able to hold my left arm straight up in the air. My right arm would stay up only when my elbow was resting on the bed, and then for just a second or two, but it was progress.

In order for Glenn to continue working, Madelyn and Beanie were kind enough to drive us down to Virginia and stay for the next two weeks while Gary and Janet were gone. Beanie was able to lift me while Glenn was at work, and Madelyn did the cooking and cleaning. I continued doing my daily exercises with their help.

Madelyn just could never quite understand why progress was so slow. Many times she would call and ask: **"Can you walk yet?"** I wished many times that I could have just jumped up and walked as appears to be possible on the TV shows, but healing takes time and revitalizing muscles cannot be done overnight. On my last visit to Dean, he told me that by September I would be up on the walker. I just grinned. I was really saying to myself: "No way. That just couldn't be possible." I was optimistic, but that just seemed out of reach as I looked at my present condition.

I was so thrilled with my progress that I shared it with several other ALS patients whom I had come to know. Three of them tried my suggestion by going to Dean, but none saw much of a change and soon stopped going to him. I often thought they should have given him more of a chance, but they seemed to be looking for immediate improvements. It may be that since I was completely paralyzed, it was easier to see each little improvement, such as moving a finger. Those whom I encouraged to try this nonconventional way of healing were all more mobile than I was when I first began; and even if they had experienced a similar improvement, it probably would not have been significant enough for them to get very excited. I wanted so much to be able to help other ALS patients, because I knew what they were going through.

The two weeks with Madelyn and Beanie went by rather quickly. Soon we were heading back to the city, picking up Janet and Gary at the airport on the way. Unfor-tunately, I had no major accomplishments to report to them. Madelyn was sure that with all the exercising I did, by the time Janet and Gary returned I would be able to show them great changes, but it just didn't happen. Little by little, progress was made, but someone who was with me day in and day out could see little happen. By the end of June, though, I was able to cross my legs at my knees and turn myself on the shower bench.

Chapter 18

Dean – Summer 1986

By the middle of July Debbie Meade had not yet written the article she had planned. When she came back from our New York trip, her research began. She decided if she were going to write an article on me that she should be sure of the facts before it went to print. In an inter-view with my Roanoke neurologist, she asked him if I had been diagnosed as having ALS. He assured her that I was. Then she wondered if he had ever had an ALS patient who improved. He said that he hadn't, but he did have a patient who hit a plateau and had remained there. He was monitoring that particular patient.

She then wanted his comments on why I was showing improvement. He would not comment on that, because he had not seen me for a year and a half. Debbie told me that she could tell that at that point he was ready to show her the door, but she continued to ask questions. As he somewhat abruptly continued to answer her questions, he finally told her he thought she would be doing a great disservice to the average person if she printed an article about my remarkable improvement. His reasoning was that it would give many patients false hope. Before she left, he made it clear he was quite interested to learn the price I was paying for my "treatment." She said that it was $750 a trip. He just rolled his eyes! It was interesting to see on the copy of my medical records, which I later got from his office. He had a written comment that I was seeing a psychic healer in New York at $750 a visit. It must have made quite an impression on him!

Debbie next tried to interview Dr. Wooten from the University of Virginia hospital, but he refused. He, too, had not seen me in a year and a half and refused to com-ment on my case. Since the two doctors who diagnosed me earlier did not satisfy Debbie's inquisitive mind, she began more research. She began calling the country's experts on ALS, all of whom said that if I were improving, I had never had the disease in the first place.

One Monday afternoon, in the middle of July, soon after Glenn brought me back from New York, the phone rang. It was Debbie. Her voice was filled with excitement. She would not tell me over the phone just what she wanted to talk to me about, but she wanted to see me immediately, if possible. I agreed to talk with her, and about ten minutes later her car came buzzing up the driveway, with the photographer close behind her. Since the weather was hot, Glenn had put me into a lawn chair so we could visit outside in the backyard. Both Gene and Debbie remarked that they could see a lot of improvement in my movements since last time they had seen me.

Then came the whole reason for coming to see me! Debbie told me she had talked with doctors from all over the country and that there was a good possibility that I didn't have ALS. All neurologists who had not seen me said that if I were improving, I definitely did not have it, since no one ever improves with that disease. A Mayo Clinic doctor suggested that it was chronic inflammatory neuropathy. She had already received permission to travel with me and the photographer to the Mayo Clinic, so I could be re-examined to determine if that is what I indeed did have. The doctor with whom she talked had been very nice to her. He seemed to give her the im-pression that if it were inflammatory neuropathy, it could be treated with medication. He said he would be glad to look at my records to see if I had been tested for it.

My first reaction was that I definitely did not want to go. I hated the idea of going through all the testing again, since I had already been through a lot. Debbie tried to convince me that I would only have to be tested for that one thing. Well, I knew better than that. I had been this route before! But she was convinced that I didn't have ALS and that I should try to find out just what I did have. She said that she would surely like to know what she had if she were in my place.

Soon her enthusiasm spread to Glenn, Gary and Janet. They, too, seemed encouraged, thinking that if the condition proved to be different, perhaps my recovery could be much faster. Well, I wasn't convinced, and I was going to do a lot of thinking about this before I rushed to the Mayo Clinic. I had called there earlier, when I first was told I had the disease, and they had had nothing to offer or suggest at that time. After about an hour of discussion, Debbie and Gene left. Upon leaving, she gave me the doctor's name and phone number so that I could contact him and discuss the matter with him personally, assuring me that he was very nice to talk with over the phone.

After they left, we ate our dinner, and I had a lot of mixed emotions, the main one being that I knew I didn't want to go through any more tests. Yet, the three people caring for me seemed to have a gleam of hope that this could lead to an early recovery. The next morning, I got on the phone and talked to the doctor at the Mayo Clinic. I used the speakerphone, since I still could not hold the receiver, and Gary was there with me to hear the whole conversation. After hearing the doctor's reaction to my questions, I think Gary then began to think, too, that it surely didn't sound as good as Debbie made it sound.

I asked the Mayo doctor if the disease had been fairly recently diagnosed, or if it were something for which tests were normally run in a case like mine. His answer was that it had been known about for the past five to ten years. I then asked about the medication, and for that the answer was that the results depended on the patient, the severity of the case and other different factors.

My last question, which I had to ask hurriedly because it did not seem as though he wanted to talk with me, was whether or not he would look at my medical records from UVA to determine if I had been tested for chronic inflammatory neuropathy, and if he thought I should have further tests. His answer was that he would not look at my records unless I became his patient. Then he said that he certainly was not looking for any new patients!

Oh, how I wished that Debbie had been there to hear that whole conversation, but she wasn't. Nor did she seem to believe what I told her had happened. I then talked to Irmtraut, my physical therapist, who told me that if she were in my place she would not go out to the clinic for more testing. She said I would just end up being their guinea pig, and the testing they would put me through would not prove anything, since my situation was improving and perhaps the stress would even slow down my recovery. She had seen many patients through her many years of working, and she believed that I did have ALS. At least she saw many of the symptoms in me that she had seen in other ALS patients. Well, that was all I needed to hear! After all, she had been the person who had been working with me more than anyone else in the medical field.

I remained curious about one thing, though: Did UVA test their ALS patients for inflammatory neuropathy? I called my doctor at UVA, and he assured me that the spinal tap results for that disease were much different from those for ALS. This gave me a feeling of relief. I also felt that I would not have to go to the Mayo Clinic to prove anything to anyone. I was satisfied with the answers from the people that I felt knew the most about my case.

When I reported back to Debbie, she certainly did not agree with my conclusion. She did not seem to trust anything that my UVA neurologist might say. Because she had talked to so many other doctors who had convinced her that I didn't have the dreaded disease, she tried over and over to convince me to go to the clinic for more tests. I could tell from our conversation that she was quite upset with my decision. It was obvious she wouldn't change my mind, and I wouldn't change hers!

I remembered what Dean had told me months before this happened: they would say I had been misdiagnosed. I decided to call Dean and tell him what had happened. His reaction was that, sure, those doctors who had seen me would say that I had Lou Gehrig's Disease and those who hadn't seen me would say I didn't have it. He continued that if I were to be tested at this point, the results would not be the same as they were when I was first tested in January of 1985. Besides, it wouldn't prove too much, no matter what the results were. He didn't think I should go through all the testing if I didn't want to, but if I did, it would be fine with him.

On July 24, Gary and I started up the pike alone. Janet had flown up to Connecticut the Saturday before to visit her family, and Glenn had to go to Blackstone, VA, on business. We made good time, going about 65 to 70 miles an hour—the usual speed for Gary in a 55 miles-per-hour zone. I often warned him that if he ever got a speeding ticket I would not pay the fine for him! Everything went fine until "Captain Video" in a white car clocked us going 70 miles an hour. That turned out to be quite an expensive trip for Gary—$82.50. I guess you learn through your own experiences!

The next day, which was a Friday, we went into the city for a 1:30 appointment with Dean. The traffic was terrible. What a difference between weekday and Sunday traffic. When we got to Dean's office, Janet was waiting for us. I went to the bathroom, and Janet and Gary left with Beanie's car to go do some business, the whole reason for making the appointment on Friday. Beanie put me on the table when Dean was ready for me, and then he and Madelyn left to walk around for the next two hours. The whole time Dean worked on me, we were discussing Debbie's approach to writing the article. He wanted me to either stop the article or ask her if she would give it to me to read before publishing it. I could understand his dissatisfaction with her emphasis on the misdiagnosis. This had happened to him many times before. It must be very frustrating to someone who has performed many miracles, but nothing he can say or do will convince someone who doesn't believe.

Since Dean was so upset, I was beginning to wonder if I would get much from our session together. But that night when I got into bed, I felt my lower arms and legs do much twitching, which had always been a good sign. Then when I returned to Virginia, I lifted my right foot up from the knee while lying on my stomach. That was something I really didn't think would happen for a long time. As I continued to exercise, I could feel my back gaining strength so that standing on my knees in front of a chair was getting a bit better. On July 30, I stood against the wall with Janet holding my knees and Gary letting me go at the shoulders for the first time since this had all begun. I only stood for a second, scared to death, but I felt like it was the beginning of getting back on my feet.

During the months of May and June, I was troubled with a vaginal odor that was about to drive me bonkers. I was sure it was a yeast infection, so I had Janet douche me. My sitting constantly created just the right condition for the yeast to subsist. Bathing didn't do much for my problem. I finally decided to call Dr. Boatwright, and he agreed to phone in a prescription for me. It was a cream that had to be inserted vaginally each day for a week. Glenn was the one elected to do the "honors." The odor disappeared within two days. Glenn did it faithfully, but after I finished the treatment I started with a vaginal itch that nearly drove me crazy. Especially when I couldn't scratch it! I was sitting outside enjoying the summer sun when I just couldn't stand the itching any longer. I told Gary to get me to the phone, because I was going to call the doctor. I told him my problem; he again called in a prescription. Can you imagine the joy it gave Glenn to know that again he would have the chore that no one else in the family wanted to do?

Again the odor reappeared after completing that spate of treatment. I decided that I had fooled around long enough with this embarrassing problem; so, I had Glenn take me down to the doctor's office to be examined. We went directly into an examining room, where Glenn undressed me and positioned me on the table. The doctor examined me and confirmed that I still had the yeast infection. He then asked Glenn whether he had been bothered with it?

He just grinned and told him he hadn't because we hadn't been doing anything. He was quick to add, not because the desire wasn't there, but because it was too much trouble. I then told the doctor that it wouldn't be long before Glenn's tongue would be hanging out from exhaustion! The doctor just laughed.

The yeast infection finally did clear up, and a month later we were able to have intercourse for the first time in more than a year. I believe someone once said that there are 101 positions in which love can be made. Well, Glenn and I often laughed about that, because there was only one way in which we could perform due to my muscle weakness.

By this time August was upon us, and it was again time to go to New York to see Dean. This time, Glenn and his parents went into the city with me. When we arrived in his office, I had the opportunity to meet a couple who had come to Dean because someone had told them about me and my fantastic improvement. The husband had been stricken with ALS, causing much weakness in his arms and affecting his speech quite a bit. I was so hoping this would be another person who would improve and share my wonderful feeling. But, as time passed, the couple decided it was too expensive for nothing, and after only a couple of visits decided to quit the treatments. Within the next year, the man passed away.

After they left the office, Glenn put me on the table, and it was time for my two-hour treatment once again. During the treatment, I meditated, and Dean had me turn on my side so that he could work on my spine. This was a dream come true. I didn't think that I would ever be able to do that, when I first went into his office in December of 1985. When he got finished working on me, he wanted to see me crawl on my hands and knees if it would not tire me too much. Well, I had Glenn put me on the floor on my knees, and I proceeded to the wheelchair in the waiting room on my hands and knees a few steps, and then the rest of the way on my elbows and knees. Everyone, including a client spectator, applauded my amazing accomplishment.

We then started back to Pennsylvania. While driving home on Rt. 24, just outside New York City, we watched a car ahead of us barely miss having a rear-end collision with a parked car in the third lane. Glenn slammed on his brakes and stopped just in time. There wasn't a person around the car. It just sat there in the passing lane. Wow, talk about shaky knees! We arrived in Virginia safely the next day, and by evening I could tell that once again I was stronger. I could lift my left leg up from the knee when lying on my stomach. My left arm and fingers seemed a tiny bit stronger. I could now eat with a fork and spoon. At times, it became quite frustrating, but practice makes perfect.

Fall seemed to be in the air the end of August when Janet and Gary put me in the car to go back up north. They decided to stay in the city with a friend Sunday night so that they could take their portfolio around to different art directors the next day. Perhaps they could get a job, do it in Virginia and send the completed project to New York. They really were not very optimistic, but they wanted to give it a shot.

I spent two hours with Dean. He was so excited about his past week, he could hardly wait to tell me about it, but first he wanted to know what progress I had made. The most important changes were that my left leg lifted up from the knee when I was on my stomach, and I seemed to be able to go much longer when on my hands and knees. He, of course, expressed his pleasure, and then began to tell me of his luck.

Paramount Pictures had found out about his script and wanted to talk with him and possibly strike up a deal. He had met with them the previous Thursday, and they had been really quite receptive. He left the script with them, and they planned to give it to Jeff Bridges to read, perhaps giving him Dean's role in the movie. He also left with them the article Debbie Mead had written in November (before I had seen Dean), along with the tapes we had made of my progress. For the next two weeks, he was going to Florida, where he would be treating the vice-president of some actor's guild and his mother. He hoped this new acquaintance would help in the search for good actors and actresses. He was still talking about my playing myself in the movie, and in TV appearances. He then suggested possibly Gary could shoot the still photos for his movie. He had already talked to Vestron about the movie, so whichever company came up with the best deal would most likely get the job. He then asked me about my book, and certainly had greater hopes for it than I! He even went so far as to say it would make a good movie. I certainly wouldn't go that far. He worked on me continually—on my legs, arms and back—until we got into about a half hour of meditating before finishing. I felt good, and I was looking forward to seeing what great things would happen the next two weeks.

After that Gary put me into Beanie's car, and I was in Madelyn and Beanie's hands for the next 24 hours. I had not stayed with anyone but Glenn and my children since I became totally dependent on someone for care, but I was confident that things would be fine. When we arrived at Madelyn & Beanie's house, Beanie put me on the floor to do some exercises. To my surprise, I was able to get on my hands and knees myself and sit up by myself. Before, someone always had to put me in that position before I could crawl. What an accomplishment! This meant that now I could do some floor exercises without someone assisting me all of the time.

Madelyn and Beanie put me to bed, and I slept well. The next morning, Beanie took me to the bathroom before he left for work in the morning, came home for lunch, performed the job again and then again when arriving home after work. That evening, Gary and Janet came back from NYC by bus with a job! They were so excited, but they had to come up with an idea for the picture. This meant that their work had to start immediately, and both Janet and Gary were drawing ideas in the car on the way back to Virginia. The photograph was completed after many long hours, and it was a real success. They continued to receive jobs from New York, not monthly, but often enough to keep them busy.

In two weeks, I was back in Dean's office for another two hours of treatment. We talked about some ideas on how we could get me up on my feet, much like a walker for children. We discussed all kinds of things, but none seemed to be adaptable to the space we had available in our house. Dean said that he would leave the designing up to my family. He said he knew we could come up with something. We got back to Virginia at 5:00 the next day. Gary made the dinner, because Janet was up at Mountain Lake as an extra in a movie called *Dirty Dancing*. Gary also told us that he had called the art director in NYC, to whom he had sent his picture that they had worked on for five days and nights, and the art director was impressed!

After returning home from this trip, I found that I could stand on my knees in front of the couch for three minutes instead of the usual minute. September 16 was the most exciting day of my life, I thought then! Gary came up with a fantastic idea to install a wire cable the full length of our hall. He would fasten a cable to the rafters in the attic, bracing the rafters. On the cable he would put a pulley with a mountain climbing rope, which attached to a harness. Together he and Glenn got it installed, and I was in business. They put me on the floor, put my legs through the mountain climbing gear and buckled it around my waist. Gary then held me up to the cable, while Janet hooked the rope to the harness. The cable was strong enough to hold my weight, so I could just hang there with no fear of falling. They then placed the walker in front of me. It was the one with wheels and arm crutches that I had used before going to the wheelchair. Luckily, it was still in the attic. At one point we had nearly given it to a person with whom Irmtraut was working and who needed one like it, but for some reason that exchange had never materialized. What luck!

Anyway, my first time up on this apparatus, I stood on my legs eight seconds. They turned blue and blotchy. Mary, my neighbor, happened to come over just as we tried it for the first time. She couldn't believe how awful my legs looked. Well, this became a daily routine, and I even sometimes did it twice a day. Gradually I became able to stay up nearly an hour at a time. I felt like a monkey in a cage, going back and forth in the hall, but I knew I had to do it. The only person who could strengthen my legs would be me. No one could do that for me.

Chapter 19

Dean ~ Fall 1986

I was with Dean for another two hours on October 4. By then, I was able to sit up in the middle of the floor, open the car door with two hands and get up on my knees in front of the couch by myself for 12 minutes. Oh yes, and flush the toilet. One time I stood at the walker with the cable's support for two minutes.

Because Dean had a cold on October 18, I did not see him again until November 1. During that month I began to take some steps with the walker when on the cable, and on October 21 the big day came. Gary lifted my butt off of the wheelchair, since I could not yet get up myself, and I stood at the walker with him following behind me with the wheelchair. I took my first step without the aid of the cable. No one will ever know the feelings I had at that time. The joy I experienced made the tears fill my eyes, and I could not say a word. If I had tried, I think I would have begun to cry, and then I wouldn't have been able to walk another step.

I continued this step routine daily, until soon no one had to follow me around with the wheelchair. I could go from room to room with the walker by myself. This was making the lifting that Gary and Glenn did almost non-existent, and the bathroom chore was also made easier. Only one person had to be with me. Janet and Gary also bought me an early Christmas present, a rowing machine, which I began using each day. After two weeks of using it I could see improvement in my arms. I began to cross stitch, open the car door with one hand and pick up a glass with one hand and drink—not easy, but possible.

November 15 came quickly, and this time Glenn drove me up to Pennsylvania. We left about 8:00 in the morning. It was raining and the bridges on the interstate were icy, making driving very hazardous for the first hour and a half. We saw many accidents and were fortunate that nothing happened to us on the way. The next morning when we got up and left for New York with Madelyn and Beanie, the roads were clear and we were able to make my 1:30 appointment in plenty of time. I had learned to do two things in the two weeks since the last time I had seen Dean: (1) 20 sit-ups without Gary pushing my head forward; and (2) crawl up on the sofa by myself. When I did the sit-ups I kept my hands in front of me, since I could not put them behind my head very easily yet.

I decided to have Dean work on me for nine treatments and give my tenth treatment to Glenn. His shoulder had been bothering him for years. About twelve years before, he had pulled on a lawn mower string trying to start it. He yanked and yanked on it every time he mowed the yard, until finally he ruined his right shoulder. It got so bad that he decided to go to the doctor. He was referred to a specialist in Roanoke, who gave him a shot of cortisone and that seemed to help for a while. After about six weeks when the pain came back, he received another shot that did nothing, so he went down to Dr. Boatwright, who said he had adhesions and the only thing that would help that would be exercise. Even though he exercised it, it continued to bother him if he moved it a certain way. Recently, though, his shoulder had begun to hurt him a lot, especially at night in bed. I'm sure lifting me aggravated it considerably. So, I decided if Dean could help me, he could help Glenn.

Glenn was sure Dean helped me, but I don't think he was convinced that Dean could help his arm. After our treatments, I thought that Glenn was able to sleep a little better without waking up with pain in his shoulder. He thought maybe it was a little better, but not a whole lot. I saw a small change in my strength. Not much, but I did notice that I could walk the length of the cable in 18 steps, and until then it had taken me 32. The following week I was able to pull my tampon out myself, which probably doesn't seem like much of an accomplishment, but, boy, that was excitement for the whole family!

On November 19, I got out of bed for the first time and walked to the bathroom. Gary also forced me to walk with the plain walker, no wheels or handles. He put me on the cable and then followed behind with the wheel-chair. Then he decided I could do it without being hooked up to the cable. I hated every minute of that maneuver. We had many arguments over what he thought I should do and what I wanted to do! My back would hurt when I did that, but I figured the more I exercised the better it would become.

A few weeks prior to this, I had been waking up nearly every hour at night with either my hips, shoulders or right knee hurting. After coming back from Dean the last time, my knee had been much better. I was sure it would be a while before all the pain went away, and my joints and muscles get used to the strain I put on them when I walked. The last time I had worked with Dean, he had told me that

I would go from the walker to the cane in a few months and eventually be off the cane. I knew I would be off of the walker at some point, but in a few months? I was doubtful.

The weekend after Thanksgiving, Glenn was headed for New Orleans for agronomy meetings, and Gary and Janet took me to Cincinnati, Ohio, for the weekend to visit Paula and Russ. Having started on our mini-vacation, we had traveled an hour when we discovered we had no brakes. We returned home—about 60 miles—without brakes over some hilly terrain. Not a very good feeling, to say the least! Glenn and Gary finally found the trouble: a broken belt to the vacuum pump that worked the brakes. After fixing that, we again started to Cincinnati, leaving at 2:00 in the afternoon. We arrived at Paula and Russ' by 9:00. While I was there, I helped roll Christmas cookies into balls. Gary and Janet taught me how to crawl down the steps backwards on my hands and knees. I crawled up the stairs, too, but Gary had to help me by lifting my one knee onto the next step. That knee just would not budge when I tried to lift it. While I was there I practiced walking on the walker with the wheels and arm rests.

Paula and Russ treated us to brunch at a revolving restaurant. It surely did feel good to be able to eat and drink everything myself, even though they did have to take me in the wheelchair. We left Cincinnati on Monday morning and traveled home in rain most of the trip. By 4:30 that evening, we had arrived at home safe and sound, with no more brake problems. Thursday night, just after midnight, Glenn arrived home from his trip. Saturday morning we were both back on the road again, headed for New York.

Sunday found us in a city filled with many Christmas lights and shoppers. My appointment was at 1:30. Frances

Podbereski, a friend of Madelyn's and mine from Bangor, went in for her usual half-hour treatment for arthritis. Before I went in for my treatments, I gave Dean a box of chocolates as an anniversary gift. It was December 7, exactly a year from the day I had first gone to see him. What a difference a year had made.

While I was in for the two hours with Dean, everyone else went up to Macy's to do some Christmas shopping. I did not get to go Christmas shopping, which did not bother me in the least. I still did not like being in the wheelchair among people. Before we left, though, Beanie did drive me around the city, so I could see the city lights.

The next morning Glenn packed the car, including a Christmas tree from his father's farm. After we got home, I saw no improvement, but by Tuesday I started my period. On many occasions that would be a time when I would show slight weakness for about three days to a week before I would see any change. This often caused me to feel depressed. It happened nearly every month, and I knew that it did, but I still did not feel very optimistic during this time. After we were home for a few days, Glenn's shoulder showed some improvement. It improved much in the same manner as I did, very slowly. After a week or so, I was able to stand a bit better when hooked on the cable. I started walking part of the time with the armrests removed. This made me feel very insecure, and my hands and feet would sweat profusely.

On December 15, I began stepping on books while on the cable. This, too, did not come easily, but then nothing did. Before going to New York again, I was kept very busy with all of the Christmas hubbub. I managed to address cards and insert a Christmas letter that I had typed on the computer. At this time, I began crawling on my hands and knees up the steps, not just down. I also began getting up from the table to the walker without someone giving me a boost. This made it easier for me to walk, because someone did not have to stop what he or she was doing to come and lift me to a standing position.

All four of us traveled to Pennsylvania in a very loaded car. With all the Christmas gifts, winter clothing, plus the wheelchair and walker, not another thing would fit. Sunday morning, we got up early. I put on my own make-up, and with everyone ready we were on the road by 9:00 headed for the city once again. We dropped Janet and Gary off at their friend's office to spend the day with him. They then planned to go to Connecticut the next day, where they would spend a week with Janet's family. I got in for my treatments about noon. Dean and I talked about my improvements since last time, about his movie plans and what we were planning for our Christmas vacations. While I was in there I also had to meditate with the light going around my body for about 45 minutes.

During my treatments, Madelyn, Beanie, and Glenn went to a restaurant for lunch. Glenn got back just in time to get his treatment for his shoulder. As we were about to leave, Rochelle gave me a small gift-wrapped box as a Christmas present. After I got in the car I immediately opened it to find a beautiful gold chain with a gold heart on it, a gift that so beautifully reflected the love that both Dean and Rochelle show toward everyone they encounter. I then ate a few carrot sticks, bologna and an apple for my lunch. We arrived at Glenn's parents' home by 5:00, and by 5:30 everyone was sitting around the supper table for our annual Buss Christmas get-together.

While we were in Pennsylvania, Glenn decided to call a fraternity brother of his who was a neurologist in Reading, PA. When he had heard about me, he had taken the time to write Glenn a letter suggesting that I should have a new test run, which had not been available when I was diagnosed in 1985. It is called the "nuclear magnetic resonance test." After talking with him, we learned that he himself had had a male patient who was diagnosed as having ALS. When the patient began losing control of his bowel, which is never lost when one has ALS, the neurologist decided to run the NMR test and discovered that his patient had a surgical lesion. After surgery, the man had improved remarkably.

After Glenn's conversation with his fraternity brother, we decided that since my improvement was coming along there was no need at that point to have further testing. The next thing on the agenda was to go up to Madelyn and Beanie's, where she was hosting an open house from 2:00 to 4:00 and from 7:00 to 9:00. About 40 people visited. I sat in a chair while everyone was there. I only walked with the walker when just a few people were around. We all had a good time. I'm sure some that attended the party were still pretty doubtful that I would ever get back to normal. Glenn and I spent the night at Madelyn and Beanie's, left the next day to spend that night at the Buss' and left for home on Christmas Day.

On Friday, Glenn helped me clean. I told him what to do, and he did it! I did run the vacuum cleaner while I was on my hands and knees. We got everything pretty well in order for Paula and Russ to stay in the back bedroom. The next day, December 27, before I went to the office with Glenn to help him with some work on the computer, he put me up on the cable to exercise as I did every morning. I decided to let go of the walker and see if I could walk without it. I placed the walker a foot or so in front of me and took a couple of steps. Soon I was walking from one end of the hall to the other without the walker, but knowing that I was on the cable and would not fall. Then

I began to wonder just how long it would be before I would be able to walk without my security blanket.

I also found that I was closer to getting my lobster dinner, which Gary and Glenn said I could have when I could wipe my own butt! I wasn't quite good enough for my dinner, though, because it wasn't white glove clean. Another new accomplishment was that I could lift the phone receiver with one hand. What progress I made this time!

On Sunday morning, Glenn went to church and I stayed at home by myself, something that I was able to do for short periods since I could get around by myself. While he was gone I made our bed for the first time. It wasn't a fast process, because I had to do it on my hands and knees. Paula and Russ came that afternoon to spend a few days, and on Monday night Glenn got dinner while they went up to Roanoke to pick Janet and Gary up from the airport. While they were gone, I washed some dishes with the walker close at hand.

Our Christmas was great. We opened our gifts that evening, with clothes being a major part of my gifts, much nicer than last year. What a difference it makes when you feel that life is just beginning rather than ending! I showed Gary and Janet how I could walk, they smiled a smile of joy and then began to chuckle. It was funny to see me walk. It was like I had my eye on my destination and made a beeline for it. If anything got in the way, I would have to stop.

By the following week, I was able to stand from a sitting position when on the bed with barely any help from the walker. I was also able to stand when sitting on the one end of the couch, by placing one hand on the arm of the sofa and the other on a pillow to help to give me a boost.

Chapter 20

1987 - Happy New Year!!!

On New Year's Day, a friend called to tell me of two former football players for the San Francisco 49ers who were part of a CNN news article. They, along with a deceased teammate, had ALS. Glenn then taped the program for me, so I could write to one of the gentlemen to let them know what action I taken and that I hoped they would try it so they, too, could experience what I had experienced. I soon heard from him, requesting the tape I had of myself throughout my recovery. It wasn't too long after that that we heard on the news that one of those gentlemen had died. The one to whom I had written viewed the tape and returned it, enclosing a letter basically telling me thanks, but no thanks. This was always disappointing to me. I continued to hope that someone else would just give it a try as I did and just maybe they would see some improvement, too. I soon found out that you could not dwell on other people's problems, lest you get yourself into a state of depression. As the saying goes, I figure I can lead a horse to water, but I can't make it drink.

On January 10, Glenn drove me to Pennsylvania, even though he was very busy with his classes. He wanted to go, not only to take me, but to have his shoulder worked on, since it hadn't seemed to improve much since last time. When we started the winter weather was very threatening, but we were very fortunate to just have foggy conditions until we got to Hamburg, about an hour away from our destination. There we hit rain and drove in it the rest of the way. Sunday and Monday turned out to be good traveling days, so our trips to the city and back to Virginia were fine.

When we went to Dean's, his office was full. While waiting, I met a dentist who practices in the city. He was aware of my recovery and wanted to talk to me about it, since he knew of someone with ALS. He wanted to know if I would talk with the victim's wife. Of course, I told him I would love to, so Glenn gave him our phone number.

My, how I wish everyone could get better! I gave the videotape we had made of my progress on January 8 to Rochelle. I then demonstrated to her how I could get up from the wheelchair myself. Everyone is always excited over my new tricks!

Dean then worked on me for two hours. He told me that Debbie Mead had called to tell them that she hoped the article would be out in January. After discussing the situation, we decided if it hit the press by April it would be lucky. When we discussed the movie, Dean said he was planning to go to LA on Monday, so further develop-ments would get under way. He was also planning on doing a talk show in the LA area while he is there the next week. I told him I was typing with my fingers now, all except my little finger. I had walked to the car with the walker three times in the past two weeks, and I was walking on the cable without the walker. My groin pull, which I had had a couple of months, was still bothering me. It woke me up hurting about every hour at night. During the day, it only hurt when I moved it a certain way, but at night it was a killer. I stressed that I would love to sleep all night!

Dean said he would work on it, and speed up the healing. By the next Tuesday, it was still hurting a lot at night. Gary thought I might be straining it all of the time when I was exercising. When I got home Monday night, I had given myself a shower, sitting on the bench, even washing my own hair. I got myself dressed, too. As long as the clothing was lightweight, I could put it on and off. And I could make the bed when on my hands and knees. I had done that for the past two weeks. After getting back from Dean's I noticed standing was a bit easier, as was making the bed. I looked forward to making big strides the next four weeks. Since I would only be seeing Dean once a month, I would have to work extra hard! I hoped to have enough energy to work on the cable twice a day.

Chapter 21

Lobster At Last!

It was now Feb. 10. A month had passed, and so much had happened. After my last trip to Dean's, I had become able to wipe my rear end. I earned my lobster dinner on my 45th birthday! I started walking with the walker with no arm supports or wheels, and on January 23 I took my first steps in the house without any walker. I walked from the sofa to the table, shaky and scared, but I accomplished it!

Another step was to go to the DMV to have my driver's license renewed. It was the first time I had gone out of the house without the wheelchair. And it looked like it would be a permanent way of transportation for me! Wow, I even went on an overnight trip to Williamsburg with Glenn, without the wheelchair and walking into three different restaurants. What a feeling!

Even though I saw pity on some faces when people saw someone so young on a walker, I felt a sense of rejoicing. Another thing that I tried and accomplished was to put my contact lenses in and out of my eyes. And I began to cook a little in the kitchen, with assistance with the pans and handling hot dishes. I made chili, meatloaf, and chocolate cake, and even peeled potatoes. It took me 45 minutes to peel seven potatoes! But I did it. I had been unable to do that before I went into the hospital. Now all I needed was patience, because everything I did, of course, went slowly. I had never liked to poke around when I did any job, but I realized I was going to learn to be satisfied with taking my time and getting done what I could.

Janet and Gary drove to Pennsylvania, since Glenn had to go to Michigan for a seed certification meeting. We took Mary Jane McMillion along and dropped her off at the Midway Diner, where she met a friend. We went on to Glenn's parents' house, changed our clothing and went out to dinner. Our party included Mom, Pop, Paula, Russ, Gary, Janet, Madelyn and Beanie, who treated all of us to a scrumptious meal.

Chapter 22

A Walking Party??

The next morning, I got myself ready with Janet's help. We had brunch at 10:30 and were off to New York by 11:15. I walked into Dean's with the walker and took a few steps for him. Of course, he was delighted. He suggested that I write to the *Today Show* as soon as I arrived home. This would give him publicity just in time for his movie. He told me of his movie, and it seemed as though things were beginning to come together. He hoped to go to LA that week to talk to several people about the production. I asked him if he would like to come to my walking party, and to my surprise he said he would not miss it for the world! So, we decided Rochelle had better call me to make the final arrangements so I could make the plans for it in either April or May. I hoped to be walking full-force by that time.

When we got back to Virginia. I found that I was a wee bit stronger, and walking by myself came a little more easily. I hoped it would improve a lot over the next month.

On March 7, Gary and Janet again drove to Pennsylvania, since Glenn was too busy to take the time from his class work. On Sunday morning, they got up and drove the car to the bus station at 6:45, left the car there and took a bus into the city. They arrived there by 9:00 and began their daylong search for housing. I was able to wash and dress myself. Wow, what a feeling! By 11:00, Madelyn and Beanie had arrived, and off we went for my 2:00 appointment. We got there on time and found a parking space. I walked in with the walker, but put it aside after I got inside. When Dean came from his office he could hardly believe that I was standing in Rochelle's office for my first time. I had never been able to go in there, since the door was too narrow for both the wheelchair and the walker. After I discussed with Rochelle the newspaper article about me that had been published February 15, the letter to the editor that Dean had submitted and the letter that Ed Mitchell had written, it was time to go into Dean's office for my two hours.

Before going in, though, I did meet a very attractive girl who had just come out of his office. She told me she had had MS for four to five years and was close to being in a wheelchair before coming to see Dean. This was her fifth time there, and she said she had improved almost immediately after seeing him the first time. She still walked slowly and with a limp, but she was able to walk the streets without any assistance!

I then spent two hours with Dean, and by the time I was finished everyone was back at the office and ready to go, including Janet and Gary. Frances Podboreski still continued to come with us, receiving two treatments, but not seeing any more signs of improvement. I went into the bathroom myself, and then we were off for Pennsylvania, where we ate supper at Perkins. The next day we headed back to Virginia, where I saw no great improvement, but I steadily got better at walking.

On April 5, 1987, Gary and Janet left Blacksburg with the truck filled with their belongings. They headed for Pennsylvania, where they unloaded everything at the Buss' and spent the night. The next week was spent hunting for a place to live. While they were getting weary in NY looking at every avenue, Glenn and I flew to Florida for a vacation. We had planned to stop off at Sunrise where Dean had planned to treat me, but due to his father's having become very ill during that week, we canceled that stop. We visited very good friends in Gainesville, my uncle in Daytona Beach, Epcot, and my cousin in Nacomus, and then went on to Busch Gardens in Tampa.

I was disappointed that I did not get "zapped" while I was in Florida, but I certainly understood. This was the longest I had been without Dean's treatments since I began seeing him in December of 1985. Even though I had not seen him, I continued to get stronger. I could not see it on a daily basis, but over a period of a month, progress was evident.

On May 5, I had the party I had dreamed of—"My Walking Party." Glenn and I picked Dean and Rochelle up at the Roanoke Airport at 10:30 a.m. We then took Madelyn, Beanie, Dean and Rochelle to Mountain Lake, where Dean treated us to lunch. We returned to our house in Blacksburg, where Dean treated me for two hours while everyone visited in the living room. Janet and Gary drove down from New York, Paula flew in from Cincinnati and everyone was ready for the party at the Marriott by 6:30. It was a great party, with door prizes, good food and friendship. Not nearly long enough. Oh, what a great feeling to be able to stand and greet my 120 guests!

I continued to improve, not fast, but at a slow, steady pace. The only occupational therapist item left in use was the shower bench. I did not drive yet, but I could finally get up off of the floor without holding onto a chair—with a little bit of work! On May 17, Irmtraut brought a gymnastics ball over for me to exercise with. The purpose was to give me more diagonal exercise and try and strengthen those muscles that were not being used very much, which eventually should produce a more balanced walk. On May 19 and 20, I went on a business trip with Glenn and was able to help him sort his seeds for planting. I hope I will be able to continue to help him with his work, even the planting and harvesting!

My next trip to New York was scheduled for June 28, and I hoped to be much improved by then. The week of June 14, I received a phone call from Carl Harris, a gentleman from Lynchburg, Va. His wife, Bonnie, had been stricken with a nerve disease. Some doctors told her it was ALS, and one doctor in Texas told her it was Lupus. In any event, it had left her paralyzed, speechless and with many of her throat muscles weakened to the point that eating was impossible. She was being nourished through a feeding tube in her stomach. Carl had called me because Bonnie had read the article in the paper about me, and she wanted to talk with me about Dean.

On June 18, a Thursday afternoon, Carl and his daughter put Bonnie in their van with a wheelchair lift and came to visit me. I showed them the tape of my progress. They were amazed, and Bonnie was convinced that she wanted to try my method. I immediately called Dean and Rochelle in Florida, and to my surprise they were at home. I had a two-hour appointment scheduled, but since their appointment book was all filled up, I asked if I could possibly give an hour of my time so that Bonnie could get in to see him on June 28. Dean agreed to do that, and it made everyone very happy.

Bonnie was looking forward to getting started on treatments. She wanted to get her speech back more than anything else. She was then communicating using an eye chart. I knew what she was going through so far as the discomfort of the paralysis was concerned, but, thank goodness, I had never had to experience the speechlessness she was facing.

On June 26, Glenn took Friday off from work and we went to Pennsylvania. We visited with Robin and Rosanne over dinner, got a good night's sleep, and the next day we took a walk down to the woods. It was my first trip down there for two and a half years. I had to have help going down the hill and back up, but I was very proud of myself that I could do that.

The next day we went into the city. Since Gary had been home for the weekend, he rode along with us. Everyone went into Dean's office and waited till I was finished, since I only took an hour instead of the usual two. When I was finished with my treatment, Dean was kind enough to give Glenn a treatment on his shoulder. When I came out of the office, the Harrises were there with Bonnie. Bonnie had written a note to Dean and was really eager to get started. They were able to get her wheelchair through the office door and lay Bonnie on the table. My one wish was that she would improve. What a wonderful thing it would be for her. Before we left, Rochelle told me that Ann Robinson, an ALS victim from West Virginia who began going to Dean after seeing the article about me, was scheduled to come in on August 9 before my appointment so we could meet each other. I was really looking forward to that.

We went back to Gary and Janet's apartment, where we unloaded everything that we had brought up for them from Virginia. We all enjoyed having dinner with them. Janet came back from Rhode Island while we were there. We left about 7:00 and got home about 10:00. The next morning we got up and left for Holland, VA, since Glenn had a meeting to attend there the next day. We stopped in to see Frank and Jane Resides in West Chester, PA, on the way. We left their place at 2:30, in the un-air-conditioned truck. We arrived in Suffolk about 10:00 that night, both exhausted from the heat. I slept all night without waking up. I think that was the first time I had done that for three years!

Irmtraut talked to me in church the next Sunday, and she wanted to come over to show me some more exercises. The following week she showed me a lot of exercises to do with weights on my legs designed to help my muscles to develop so I could go up and down the steps better. With the extremely hot weather, exercising was not easy, but I tried to do as much as I could. I surely hoped it wouldn't be too long until I could climb the steps without holding onto the railing.

On July 14, I went down to Dr. Boatwright`s office to have him complete a medical form so that I could keep my driver's license. He was really pleased to see me, and after examining me he told me that he didn't ever want to see me without a smile on my face! He said that if I wasn't driving, it wasn't because I couldn't drive, but because I wanted to be chauffeured. Well, then I decided to try to drive while we were in Cincinnati visiting with Paula and Russ. Glenn rode with me around the parking lot. This was on July 18, and driving seemed to be very easy to do. I was quite surprised that I wasn't more nervous. Nothing seemed weak at all. I then began to drive more often, and by Thursday of that week I drove to the hair-dresser's by myself. The first step to getting out into the real world! I presumed I was improving little by little, even though it didn't seem like much to me.

Can You Walk Yet?

Chapter 23

Getting Back to a Normal Life

Life began to return to normal. Gary and Janet moved back to NYC to continue with their photography business. I started helping Glenn with the harvesting of his soybean research plots at both Blacksburg and Warsaw, VA. Paula and Russ bought a three-story house in Cincinnati, Ohio. Glenn and I spent a week out there removing wallpaper and painting a bedroom, preparing for their first baby's arrival. On June 14, 1988, Flag Day, Aaron was born. Glenn and I bought 1.75 acres of land about ten minutes from downtown Blacksburg. We cut trees and cleared the land. Construction began in February of 1989. We spent many hours making decisions on both the interior and exterior. We spent three weeks installing a slate floor in the dining room, entryway and hall. We sold our house and lot on Orchard View Lane, where we had lived for the past 20 years. Madelyn and Beanie came down and with their help and the help of friends and neighbors, we were able to move into our new house in July. Our travels throughout the year of 1990 took us to St Louis and Las Vegas for Glenn's professional meetings. And, of course, out to Ohio to see our grandson and to Pennsylvania for a family reunion.

After four years of walking again, I started joining different community groups and helping with soybean planting and harvesting. My days were busy and fulfilling. A few years earlier, I never imagined I would be able to do half of what I was able to accomplish. In 1991, we became grandparents again with Aaron's brother, Christopher, coming into the world in the car at a fire station on the way to the hospital. I was able to go to Cincinnati and help Paula and Russ with the new addition.

Also in 1991, Glenn's father suffered from a bad heart and failing kidneys. In June, he passed away and left behind a lot of good memories. Glenn's mother suffered with a severe case of shingles soon after his death, so we made several trips to Pennsylvania during the year. She suffered with the aftereffects of the shingles until the end of her life, four years later.

In July 1992, Gary and Janet left Blacksburg for a cross-country bike trip. They biked as far west as Wyoming, where they decided biking across the Rockies was a little more than they wanted to tackle. They rented a car, drove to Oregon, biked around Oregon, went into a pawn shop, bought a wedding ring, got married and flew back to NYC where they had jobs waiting. They were becoming dissatisfied with New York life and decided they would like to move back to Blacksburg and start their own photography business. They purchased an eight-room house on Main Street in Blacksburg, which needed a lot of renovations.

1993 was a busy year. Glenn and I traveled to Hawaii. This was a trip we had planned for our 25th anniversary, but for obvious reasons it had not taken place. After we returned, the Fox TV network came to our house to film 'Sightings,"a program that focuses on the unbelievable.

After that aired, people called to talk with me about my healing.

On October 4, Kate, Gary and Janet's first child, was born. It was so good to have them back in Blacksburg to give us a chance to spoil our only granddaughter.

On January 26, 1995, Glenn's mother passed away after having suffered a brain aneurism the previous November. In May of that year, Glenn and his two brothers had an auction to sell the farm machinery and household goods. A 'home' that we were used to visiting several times a year was no longer. Later that year, we traveled to Memphis and St. Louis for Glenn's professional meetings, and to Asheville, NC, where Paula and Russ had moved to start up Russ' new engineering business.

In April 1996, a portion of Glenn's farm was sold at auction. That land is now a housing development. His brother purchased about half of the farm. He still lives there and runs a truck farming business. On May 9 of that year, Cameron, Kate's brother, was born.

In 1997, I went to Pennsylvania with Janet and Gary. The reason I went along was so I could babysit Kate and Cam while Gary and Janet went into NYC to do a photo shoot. We stayed with Madelyn and Beanie. To keep the children entertained, we invited my childhood friend, Lucille, to go along when we took the children to Chuckie Cheese. It turned out to be a fun day.

In May of that year, we started building a greenhouse/ sunroom on the back of our house. We dug the footers by hand, and Beanie helped lay the concrete block foundation wall. Paula and Russ came to help us when the cement truck came to pour the concrete. We contracted with a company to put up the framework, glass and brick floor.

They finally completed the job Oct. 10. Glenn's brothers and their families came down to visit, their first visit since we had been in our new house.

In 1998, ten years after having learned to walk again, Dean Kraft contacted me to ask me to appear on some TV shows to help him promote his book *A Touch of Hope*. We appeared on *The Public Eye*, *The Maurey Povich Show* and *The View*. Being interviewed by Meredith Vieira was an exciting experience, even though it did make me a bit nervous, since it was before a live audience. *The Public Eye* crew came to the house to interview us. That was a bit less stressful.

During August and September of that year, we used a pick and shovel to cut down a bank in the backyard so that we could have a rock wall built. I would have never dreamed I would ever be able to swing a pick again! That year we also took Kate down to Asheville with us to visit her cousins. We took her to the Thanksgiving parade and to see the gingerbread houses on display at the Grove Park Inn. When we got close to home, she said she was going to run into the house just as fast as she could. She was really glad to be home!

On October 10, 1999, Dean's movie, "A Touch of Hope," aired on NBC. It did have a small segment about my healing, but no one would have recognized me. The woman playing my part had her feet up on a coffee table drinking a beer!

The spring of 2000 found us working hard to ready our yard and garden for the Blacksburg Garden Tour. About 200 people stopped by. We enjoyed it, but it was a lot of work, and we decided we would not do it again! After that event was over we started preparing for a trip to Germany,

Switzerland and Austria. That was a trip of a lifetime. They were all beautiful countries!

In 2002, Glenn turned 62 and decided to take a retire-ment package that Virginia Tech was offering to counteract a budget shortfall. He officially retired June 30, but that did not mean that his work stopped. He continued to work nearly fulltime (with no pay), so that his soybean program would not dry up. He did this for almost three years, until Virginia Tech finally found enough funds to hire someone to take his place.

I had stomach problems, which continually seemed to get worse. I went to a surgeon, who performed a lot of tests and decided to take out my gallbladder. After I recovered from that, my stomach did not seem to have improved very much. I later found out it was Irritable Bowel Syndrome, which cannot be treated easily. Anyway, then it was Glenn's turn to start seeing doctors. He started feeling tightening in his chest when we took our morning walks. He went to a cardiologist in Radford Sept. 11, 2003, to have a catheterization to check things out. When the surgical team got in there, they found four blockages. One was 99 percent closed. They immediately arranged for him to go by ambulance to Roanoke, where doctors were able to insert a stent to take care of two blockages. He returned to the hospital on Oct. 2 to have two more stents inserted to take care of the other two blockages. After six weeks of recuperating, he was good to go.

Glenn continued to work at Tech with the soybean program. In 2005, his position was finally filled, and we were able to take a ten-day river cruise up the Mississippi. In May, we went to Asheville to keep Aaron and Christopher while Paula and Russ went to a National Boy Scout Convention in Texas. We were able to get a little work done around their office building and house while we were there. We enjoyed Thanksgiving dinner at our house that year with Madelyn and Beanie and Gary's family. Paula, Russ and the boys came for the Christmas Holiday.

In June 2006, we went to Asheville to celebrate Aaron's graduation from high school. In July, Paula and Russ came up with the boys to take Aaron to Virginia Tech for orientation. At that time, Paula was concerned about Russ. He seemed to be dragging his one foot, but Glenn and I had no idea there was anything wrong. They left our house on a Thursday. The very next Saturday, Russ became ill with a bad headache. Paula took him to the emergency room, and by 12:00 that night he had been diagnosed with a brain tumor. The medical team did a biopsy and found out that he had glioma blastoma, the worst of all brain tumors. Glenn and I went to Asheville to help build a ramp, so Russ would be able to get in and out of the house. He was having difficulty walking. He was able to get into Duke, which is known for having one of the best doctors for his condition. He started chemotherapy immediately. It seemed to help for a bit, but his memory began to deteriorate, and it was getting more and more difficult for Paula to care for him.

Aaron started school here at Virginia Tech in August. He came over to our house every Sunday to have a meal with us and do his laundry. The first day of classes that year, a prisoner shot the guard who had taken him to a hospital bathroom. After that, the prisoner escaped wearing clothing that his brother had put up in the bathroom ceiling, then went on a walking trail near campus and shot a deputy sheriff. Virginia Tech was on lockdown until law enforcement officers were finally able to catch the man in some bushes very near campus.

On November 11, Paula called us to tell us that Russ had passed away. Gary and Janet picked up Aaron at his dorm and took him home. I was dealing with pneumonia at the time, but was able to recover enough to attend the funeral. There were 400 people who came through the reception line. Russ was well known throughout the community. We stayed with Paula for the week following the funeral, a really difficult time when you have lost your husband, especially at the young age of 46.

In spite of all the turmoil in his life his first year of college, Aaron was able to keep up his grades. In the fall of 2008, Christopher followed his brother and started his studies at Virginia Tech. We usually had a full house on Sundays. Gary and Janet and family, plus the boys, usually came for dinner. It was great to have everyone together. I continued to have bouts of pneumonia, so in 2009 after many tests they decided that it was due to acid and bile reflux. I had fundoplication surgery done via laparoscopy to tighten the esophagus. After the surgery, it was difficult to eat very much for a few weeks, but I was soon able to eat normally and the bouts with pneumonia stopped.

In 2011, Beanie, our dear brother-in-law, came down with bladder cancer. He had surgery in a Philadelphia hospital. My sister was suffering from dementia, so we went to Pennsylvania to be with her at the hospital during surgery. We would travel to Bangor often, because my sister was no longer able to cook. I made food to take along so they would have it. Beanie was in and out of the hospital several times. Finally, in September, he was told there was nothing else that could be done, and he ended up in a nursing home near his home. We were there when he passed away in October that same year. We stayed with Madelyn for a week after his death. She needed help with her finances. She could not do any of the paperwork herself. I hired a friend to come a few days a week to take her to the store, hairdresser, dentist, etc.

While Beanie was in the hospital, he realized that he and Madelyn did not have a have a will or power of attorney. So Beanie had me contact his cousin to acquire a lawyer, whom she recommended. Beanie wanted Gary and me to take over the responsibility of medical and financial power of attorney, but I didn't think I could handle it since I lived 400 miles away. I suggested that it would be better to have a member of Madelyn's and my extended family, who lived only 45 miles away, and who, for simplicity, I will call "William." William and our son, Gary, would together carry out that responsibility. We thought it would be a cooperative effort to see that Madelyn's finances and health issues were taken care of. I talked to the lawyer and told him that he would have to meet with Beanie at the nursing home, to which he was being transferred from the hospital, to get the necessary papers signed. We thought it was a 'dual' power of attorney, so Gary would have just as much right to do things as William did. We soon found out that Gary had no rights at all unless something happened to William.

Two years after Beanie died, William had completely taken over. He told us very little and watched our every move when we visited Madelyn via cameras he installed in her house. That is not the way Beanie wanted it, but who would have thought a member of my own family would neither let me participate in my sister's care nor communicate anything about her well-being? When he did communicate, it was to tell me what I could and could not do, and to show that he had complete control. It made our family's life very stressful, but it appeared there wasn't a thing we could do about it. Eventually, he completely isolated me from my own sister. Beanie would have been appalled if he had known what had happened. This has been a hard lesson learned in dealing with life, death and the inevitable wrinkles in life.

William would lie and go to great lengths to convince everyone that he had control and he was doing everything for Madelyn's best interest. It is amazing what power and money can do to a person, just unbelievable. I am so glad I shared the best part of our lives together, and she was not aware of everything that was going on around her.

As everyone knows, dementia can rob a person of her mind, but allow her to linger for years. It is probably hardest for the family members who watch loved ones lose their memory and require help for everything they do. My sister succumbed to a heart attack on July 24, 2016. What a blessing!

Our two grandsons from Asheville, NC, graduated from Virginia Tech in 2012. Having completed a couple of internships during his college years, Aaron received his master's in computer science and made the decision to work for Qualcom in Raleigh, NC. Christopher graduated in biology and started medical school at Chapel Hill, NC. He is now in his third year and starting his residency program. They both married. Aaron's wife is a Spanish teacher at a high school close to their home and gave birth to our first great-grandchild, Connor, born July 16, 2016. Christopher's wife is a graduate of Duke University and is now working toward a master's degree in global health. She will be going to Kenya for the summer to gather information for her thesis.

Our other two grandchildren, who live here in Blacksburg, have also decided to attend Virginia Tech. Kate is enrolled in the human nutrition, foods, and exercise program. She is a member of the university biking team and a pro team in California. Her goal is to become a Pro Biker. She is good at it, but it is not a very lucrative sport. We all worry about her, because it is a dangerous sport. She has already had two accidents while training. Training takes a lot of her time. She trains nearly every day, sometimes on a stationary bike for four hours at a time. We'll see how life works out for her!

Her brother, Cam, is in mechanical engineering and is doing an internship with a company in Buffalo, NY. He will return to Blacksburg in August to start his junior year. It is always nice to see that the grandkids are doing so well.

Thirty years after my being diagnosed with ALS, Glenn and I continue to work in the garden and yard. He stays busy with woodturning and beekeeping. I still belong to a few organizations, have lunch with friends and keep up with friends and family on the Internet and telephone. Aren't computers great, if everything works as it is supposed to work?

Healing takes courage,

and we all have courage,

even if we have to dig a little to find it.

Tori Amos

Made in the USA
Columbia, SC
20 July 2017